9-5-74

# The Story of Josh

# The Story of Josh

## Marcia Friedman

PRAEGER  PUBLISHERS
New York • Washington

Published in the United States of America in 1974
by Praeger Publishers, Inc.
111 Fourth Avenue, New York, N.Y. 10003

© 1974 by Praeger Publishers, Inc.
*All rights reserved*

Library of Congress Cataloging in Publication Data

Friedman, Marcia.
  The story of Josh.

  1. Brain—Tumors—Personal narratives.  I. Title.
RD663.F7        362.1′9′6992810924 [B]        73-21463
ISBN 0-275-19960-6

Printed in the United States of America

1824667

# Contents

# Prologue

A man, though he dies before his time,
    shall be at rest, for an honored old age
    does not depend upon length of time,
    nor is it measured by the number of one's
    years. . . . Being perfected in a little
    while, he fulfilled long years, for
    his soul pleased the Lord.
                    Wisdom of Solomon 4:7–8, 13–14

At dawn on March 1, 1973, at the UCLA Medical Center, my firstborn son, Joshua Paul Friedman, in the twenty-first year of his life, died. His death ended thirteen unendurable months of vain struggle against a malignant glioma, an incurable tumor of the brain. His one flaw was this obscene cancer. Death did not defeat him, as living had never overwhelmed him, and his year of dying was such an incredible demonstration of growth, dignity, grace, courage and personal control that an account of his struggle and victory over the ultimate loss must be told. There is nothing so lonely as the terminal illness of a young person. Someone else's agony cannot reduce the suffering, but there is some solace in knowing that one is not unique in the gray world of fear, pain and isolation. If Josh's story can serve as an example and be of help to others who must face untimely death, then it will be of inestimable value. And so the book.

Josh had a great sense of self-value, a great desire to live. He knew that he was destined to make a mark on his time. When it was determined that his death was inevitable, and he knew that time would not permit him to explore his potential to find the area where he might make his personal contribution to society, he consciously decided, I believe, to make his manner of dying tolerable and strangely rewarding to those of us who suffered his loss personally. He also hoped his experience might benefit others who suffer. Shortly before his death he asked me if I would write a book about him so that he would not have just passed through life without some tangible remembrance, and I promised him I would. And so the book.

Periodically, during the last few months of his life, as he lay wracked with excruciating pain, Josh made about six hours of tapes for us. They are heartbreaking for us to listen to—and they are heartbreakingly beautiful. He made them for several reasons. He wanted them to be sources of solace to us after his death—links with him when he was no longer with us. He wanted us to be sure (as though there could be any doubt after the agonizing months that we spent with him) that he felt only love, never bitterness. In thirteen months this incredible young man never once asked, "Why me?" He made the tapes also to take his mind off the unremitting pain. During those last weeks any activity, however placid, was physical torture. And so he talked and reminisced and, hopefully, did for a few moments forget the pain. The tapes reflect the brain damage he had suffered, particularly in the areas of communication: Some words are reversed, there is much repetition, and he gropes for words that he cannot summon to the surface. But the message is never distorted, and his logic is never faulty. Portions of these tapes, edited but not changed, will parallel my account of his illness and death. In effect, Josh is posthumously sharing in the writing of his story. And so the book.

A catastrophic illness of this sort, which bursts without warning upon a family, traumatizes all the members of the family. As in a physical explosion, the epicenter receives the greatest damage but the shock waves extend outward—cracking, damaging, threatening. The extended family, friends, acquaintances and the medical personnel involved are all affected to varying degrees. Josh's illness, and the way he dealt with it, made deep impressions on many of the people who came into contact with him during the last year. Moreover, the various ways in which other people behaved toward him affected him and us differently. There was much kindness shown toward him—and there was much needless, heedless cruelty. Ignorance of appropriate

4

behavior in the presence of the terminally ill is a problem that can and should be recognized and dealt with. And so the book.

I shall write the story of this tragedy as faithfully, as honestly as is possible. It will, however, be two personal accounts of what happened—Josh's and mine—and will therefore reflect our individual biases and interpretations. There is no intent on my part to have the book serve as a polemic against the medical profession; but by the same token, neither is it a panegyric in their behalf. Therefore, the names of the doctors involved have been changed to pseudonyms. Much of the resentment I feel concerning Josh's death (for I never was able to be as loving and gracious about it as he) does reflect a disenchantment with our medical practices, but it is not directed personally toward any of the doctors. The members of our medical profession are as much slaves to the cultural conventions of our society as are the patients and their families. I feel strongly that many of these conventions are long overdue for re-examination and, perhaps, change. And so the book.

In classical drama a tragedy was a story of a seemingly most fortunate protagonist who suffered a frightful end as the result of a single flaw. Whatever the flaw, it set in motion a series of events that, once initiated, led inexorably and irreversibly to the destruction of the central figure of the drama. The purpose of tragedies was two-fold: They were cathartic, as the viewers identified and empathized with the figures in the play. And they were educational in that they revealed some of the complex interrelationships between action and its consequences, and how the people caught up in them rose to the challenges and were destroyed, but not defeated, by them. Not every sad story of death is a tragedy. To qualify for that status it must have universality and grandeur; the protagonist must rise above mere extinction and, in losing, somehow win. I do believe that my son Josh was such a figure.

# Winter 1972

Seek not to understand what is too difficult
for you, search not for what is hidden
from you. Be not overoccupied with
what is beyond you, for you have been
shown more than you can understand.

Apocrypha, Ben Sira 3:21–23

We first learned of Josh's critical illness from Josh himself. It was a Friday evening and we had arranged to meet him for dinner at a fairly good restaurant close to our office. He had called late in the afternoon and suggested that we might enjoy his company for dinner. Of course I was delighted. In the five or six weeks since he had moved from our house to an apartment close to the university we hadn't seen him often and, although I considered that both appropriate and desirable for him, I naturally looked forward to a visit with him. Leib and I had arrived a little early for our appointment and were enjoying a cocktail, chatting about business, when Josh arrived.

I saw him as he entered and waved him over to join us. It gave me a renewed sense of pride and pleasure to see him —his long, lean body, his handsome face with that flawless, sun-tanned skin, the predictable broad smile, those big, innocent hazel eyes. He wore his thick, brown-black hair almost shoulder length with its soft wave and shiny clean vital look. Inevitably, several diners turned their heads to follow his passage through the room. He was surpassingly handsome and all his life he'd been the focal point for admiring glances from both men and women. If he was aware of the staring, he was certainly unconcerned about it.

We talked comfortably about this and that as we ate dinner. He told us about his classes, the new friends he was making, about his improving social life. We in turn were happily able to tell him that business was finally starting to pick up for us, so much so that we had just applied for medical insurance. (We'd had no coverage since Leib had left the aerospace industry some seven months before and we'd moved to Santa Barbara and started work in real estate.)

This must have been the opening in the conversation Josh was waiting for. He smiled ruefully and said, "That's good, because we may be facing some *really big* medical bills. The doctor sent me to a neurosurgeon and he thinks I might have a big problem. You know, I may not make it to my twenty-first birthday."

It was an utterly outrageous statement. He had to be joking. We started questioning him. It developed that he had been feeling ill, strange, in many ways. He'd gone to the general practitioner recommended to us and, in turn, Dr. Alexander had sent him to a specialist, Dr. Harmon. We were to call Dr. Harmon and he would be able to give us further clarification. It sounded so catastrophic, yet Josh seemed so calm that it was difficult to believe what he was saying. We finished the meal without another reference to this subject; he left for his place and we went home.

We spent the next two days in a numbed, vaguely fearful state. We had to wait until Monday to speak to the doctor. After re-evaluating, dissecting, overanalyzing the skimpy information Josh had given us, we concluded that some gross error in interpretation had occurred and we should just try to function normally until we could clarify the situation.

We did function. Leib went to the office as usual. I puttered about with household chores and spent some time at the office as well. We tried to act as if nothing had changed. But on Sunday we decided not to go to Los Angeles to the party that was being given by a friend of mine who'd recently remarried.

Finally, Monday morning I was able to contact Dr. Harmon's office and arrange an appointment with the doctor for four o'clock that afternoon. The hours dragged by. At four, we were ushered into the inner office by the receptionist and Dr. Harmon came forward from his desk to greet us with hand outstretched. We shook hands, accepted chairs pulled up before the desk as he settled himself back in his swivel chair with a broad smile. He told us that he'd seen Josh at the request of Dr. Alexander, who had discovered a disturbing degree of papilledema (pressure in the eyeballs) during his last checkup.

He said, "My examination confirmed this pressure. This was in combination with hand tremors, flickering sensations behind the eyes and in the head, brief (two- to three-second) losses of memory and occasional, brief vision loss in the right eye. Except for the fact that Josh says he has no headaches, these symptoms indicate a strong possibility that he has a brain tumor. In my opinion Josh should be immediately hospitalized for further testing."

We had been aware of Josh's nervousness during the few months he'd been with us in Santa Barbara before he moved to an apartment in Isla Vista, but he'd never spoken of any of these other problems. Logically enough, we'd attributed his general malaise to his unhappiness at having to live at home after two years away at school and to his loneliness and boredom without his good buddies at San Diego, since he hadn't yet made new friends in Santa Barbara. Dr. Harmon, and several other doctors whom we saw later, confirmed that this pattern of silence toward parents about physical problems among young adults, particularly boys, seems to be quite common.

We got back to the specific problem. "Why," I asked Dr. Harmon, "is there such a rush? And what would the tests involve?"

Dr. Harmon cleared his throat and responded, "If your son has a tumor and it's untreated, I wouldn't give him more than four or five months. As far as the tests go, we'll run some electroencephalograms, X rays, brain scans. We'll also give him an angiogram; that's a technique we use to get a dye substance to the brain to help define the location and extent of the tumor. I must tell you that this testing procedure has an element of risk—about a one in two hundred fatality rate. Surgery, if it proves necessary, obviously has a higher element of risk. But time is of the essence. Josh should be hospitalized immediately."

We were stunned. We could hardly believe what the doctor was saying. What's more, he was actually giggling as he told us these horrors. I realize now, that working as he does with such devastating physical problems, he probably adopted his excessively bright, light, and almost foolish approach as a defense. But at the time, we were much disconcerted by his manner.

We told him that we wanted another opinion. "Of course," he agreed, and then, "Naturally. Ha, ha, ha. After all, how many sons do you have? Hah, hah, hah." We sat in stunned silence, appalled by his apparent insensitivity.

When I asked him, "Who is the best man in this field on the West Coast?" there was no hesitation on his part. He said, "Dr. Stark, at UCLA."

He told us that Dr. Stark was very busy, very much in demand, and very selective in choosing his patients. But we were not to be put off, and so secured both Dr. Stark's phone number and a firm promise of cooperation from Dr. Harmon. We raced home with the telephone number.

The next hour and a half is a blur of confused telephone calls in my memory. In spite of several wrong starts, I finally reached Dr. Stark's office; they contacted Dr. Harmon, who confirmed that Josh's case was both urgent and dramatic. (Since UCLA Medical Center is a teaching hospital they lean toward difficult or interesting cases for instructional value.) We arranged for a visit on Wednesday, February 9, 1972 at 1 P.M., less than forty-eight hours away.

Within the space of one hundred minutes, we had made the first of the many instantaneous, critical decisions we would be pressured into making continually throughout the course of Josh's illness, usually at the insistence of doctors. Every new move, every new choice, would henceforth be presented to us with the time factor as a major determinant. Assuredly, time is a significant consideration; but I strongly believe, in retrospect, that too much emphasis is placed on the importance of speedy action. This isn't, of course, a medical evaluation. It is a human evaluation. There was never time enough before Josh's hospitalization and subsequent surgery for us to do any research in the literature on brain tumors. There was insufficient time for us to be made fully cognizant of the potential problems that could result from brain surgery, even if it had proved to be successful. The possibility and extent of postoperative handicaps were never adequately described. We never had a chance to evaluate the possibility of our son's survival without surgery. We were never told—it was never even suggested—that there might be alternative treatments.

Most medical thinking seems to be weighted toward a quantitative measure of survival, with little concern for the qualitative aspect of that survival. Surgical techniques, highly developed in this country, are given overwhelming pre-eminence in medical practice. We are all—doctors, patients, and families—conditioned by our social attitudes to accept almost any devastating procedure in the battle to live, in the struggle to avoid death. Death is the only recognized enemy. But we—Josh, Leib, and I—learned bitterly what most of us instinctively know is the real truth: that dying is the real terror and death can be a welcome friend.

We arrived with Josh on Wednesday at the huge UCLA Medical Center on the Westwood campus. After traversing what seemed to us miles of corridors, we found the right elevator and rode to the seventh floor to Dr. Stark's office. A nurse-receptionist led us across the hall to a small, simply outfitted, sterile little cubicle. We waited for just a few moments until the doctor came in.

Dr. Stark is cast in exactly the image I had of a neurosurgeon. He was at that time, I would guess, in his early fifties. He is perhaps five feet ten but seems much taller because of his slender build and rigidly erect carriage; not handsome, but rather distinguished-looking, with thinning gray hair, clear blue eyes and so light a complexion that it imparts an almost translucent quality to his skin. His hands, though long-fingered, seem more practical than aesthetic. His manner was grave and serious but neither grim nor patronizing. He is that rare man, a true gentleman. From that first visual contact, all of us felt we had fortunately found the very best surgeon available. That opinion was never to change.

We gave the doctor a concise but reasonably complete account of Josh's medical history. His birth, although forceps-assisted, had been well within the range of normal. There had been considerable cranial distortion, but not to a greater degree than expected under the circumstances; time and growth had returned it to near symmetry within his first year. He achieved a high level of muscular coordination and sense perception quite early. His rate of growth, of both height and weight, was very rapid and was accompanied by a truly precocious intellectual development. He had very few baby illnesses. Just before the age of three, shortly after Simon was born, he developed asthma. We had him treated with weekly injections, and within a few months it had been brought under control. He still suffered occasional attacks but responded well to medication; with the passage of time, his asthma gradually diminished in intensity and frequency. It never attained major proportions and was never so severe as to limit, for more than a day or two at a time, his normal schooling or play activities. He had his tonsils out at about six, a few simple bone fractures between nine and twelve, treatment for nasal polyps at fifteen. When he was about seven or eight he'd had some dizzy spells and we'd taken him to the doctor for that. They ran a series of electroencephalograms at that time and the readings had been negative—or, in other words, normal. The dizzy spells had not recurred.

When Josh was sixteen he suffered a convulsive seizure. He had just come home from school when it occurred. Fortunately, and quite by chance, Leib was home at the time. The seizure lasted just a few moments—perhaps thirty seconds. As soon as it stopped, and Leib had made sure that Josh was all right, he called our family doctor, who recommended immediate hospitalization to determine the cause.

The hospital doctors kept Josh there for two days while they ran a battery of tests to eliminate the various possibilities, such as diabetic coma. The electroencephalograph readout indicated a grand mal epileptic seizure. A neurologist was consulted and confirmed the findings. Our doctor, Dr. Rubin, told us the diagnosis and assured us that in most cases epilepsy could be controlled with just oral medication; barring an intractable case, Josh could live a perfectly normal life. He said that of the range of possible illnesses Josh might have had, we were lucky it was this one. His activities would be in no major way curtailed, provided he used reasonable judgment and avoided excesses of any sort. In short, moderation in all things would have to be his rule. After surviving the initial shock of the diagnosis, with the archaic stigma carried by the word "epilepsy," Josh functioned just as before. The medication, dilantin and phenobarbital, was adjusted once or twice until a balanced dosage was reached and, so far as we knew, Josh never had another seizure.

Now, Dr. Stark's questioning brought us back to the symptoms that Josh was currently experiencing. When he spoke to Josh his total concentration was focused on the boy, not only during this initial visit but through all of Josh's many visits with him, even when our son was having the greatest difficulties in communicating. It was plain that, although we might listen, we were not to participate in the dialogue. I think it was this clearly defined doctor-patient relationship, this man-to-man quality, that always gave Josh such a feeling of confidence when he saw Dr. Stark. Even during Josh's last months of decline, and despite the full knowledge that there was nothing more Dr. Stark could do for him, just having the doctor's undivided attention gave him a sense of comfort. Only when the doctor withheld information or was evasive did Josh feel anger toward him, never for his inability to provide a cure. He was the *only* doctor we encountered who gave all of his attention to Josh on every occasion that he saw him—even if just for a minute or two on hospital rounds.

I was surprised at the meticulousness with which Josh was able to describe his flickering vision, the degree of hand tremor, the mystical quality of the memory lapses. He must have been giving much thought to these symptoms without ever mentioning them to us. He also astonished us by telling Dr. Stark that he'd had two other seizures while he'd been in San Diego. He'd never told us, although we always asked how he'd been feeling—again that "keep-the-folks-out-of-it" attitude. I don't know if it was to keep the family from worrying, or to deny by the act of silence that he had a defect; perhaps a combination of both. Dr. Stark didn't seem a bit surprised that we hadn't been told and, at least, Josh now had the good sense to be completely honest with the doctor.

They went into an adjoining room for an examination. Some time later the doctor returned and, while Josh was still away dressing, the doctor told us, "All my preliminary tests indicate the likelihood of a tumor in the left hemisphere of the brain, just as Dr. Harmon told you. I strongly advise that you bring him here to the hospital as quickly as possible for extensive testing. I'll undertake the case." We tried to press for more information, but he could not provide anything more specific until they'd had a chance to conduct the tests. He was very solemn, and we were very worried, but the only possible approach would have to be one step at a time.

When Josh came back, the doctor told him what he had already told us. There was the delicate question of balancing parental authority against Josh's emerging young manhood. Josh was twenty. At that time the legislature was seriously considering granting full majority to eighteen-year-olds (which it finally did). We were legally responsible for him, but he also had medico-legal rights. For example, if he had contracted VD and had gone to a doctor for treatment without our knowledge, that doctor not only would not have to consult us for permission to treat him but could not even inform us of Josh's disease without his permission. Aside from any legal considerations, Josh was a very strong-willed, self-confident young man. We had always tried to instill in him a sense of his own worth and intelligence together with a sense of responsibility. It was *his* brain we were talking about. It was *his* person that would be subjected to the tests. *His* life was the life in danger. We could encourage, we could suggest, we could volunteer opinions, but the decision had to be his. Josh agreed to enter the hospital for testing but not, as the doctor suggested, the following day. He would come on Sunday. He wanted a few days to think about things, to prepare himself. Oh, Josh, dear heart, how wise you were. You cheated fate and gained your last four days of normalcy, pain-free, handsome, confident, bright and happy.

17

Thursday we didn't see Josh. He told us he had things to do at school, and had a date for that evening. We found out later that he had spoken to all of his instructors and had taken official sick leave from the university so that he would not jeopardize either his grade point average or his standing with the institution upon his hoped-for return. Also, in his marvelously organized way, he had actually spent the evening getting all his books, films, clothes and papers in order in his room at the apartment. He had started the pattern that would mark his last year of life. He was taking control. He was doing things *his* way, at *his* time. Within the limits of his ability to affect the course of future events, he was in the director's chair. Perhaps he suspected even then that he would never be returning to his apartment. I don't know.

Throughout the entire course of his illness, Josh always seemed to have some prior knowledge, or at least a suspicion, of what would be confirmed medically. As he told me later, and repeated on one of his tapes to us, his *brain* was the damaged part of him—*not his mind.* Maybe psychologists and philosophers will continue to argue the question of mind-brain unity or dichotomy; for me there is no doubt as to their exclusive properties. I saw their divergence in my son. Not the tumor that strangled a portion of his brain, nor the surgery that traumatized it beyond recovery, nor the cobalt that seared those physical convolutions ever touched his mind, his inner self. His mental crippling was an outward manifestation, not an inner one. Maybe the French are right to have one word for both mind and soul. Both are concepts beyond the power of either definition or understanding.

*This is September 8, 1972. My name is Joshua Paul Friedman. I was born almost exactly twenty-one years ago. My birth date is October 10, 1951 — I am almost twenty-one. What I have to say is very, very difficult for me to say—and I am also having a difficult time saying what I want to say. This is for a number of reasons and I'll try to explain some of them as I go along. One important thing that I do want to say now is extremely important. You must understand I do not have my full capabilities to say what I want to say. I'm not as smooth a talker as I used to be, and sometimes I may have to say things that are not exactly what I want to say . . . but I do have to say them. I have many things to say and I will try and get to the important things.*

*My past is very, very straight on the line. I recall my past and it must recall me, whatever that means. I was gifted as a child, as a young child, as a young child under one year old, with a memory; that is to say, with a little nudging or pushing I can remember everything that has ever happened to me . . . I do have my first memories definitely before I was one year old.*

*There was one time, I don't exactly remember exactly what home we lived in at that time, my parents were married and I was their first child, I was under one year old, and I remember. My father came over to me. I imagine he kissed me and all that, but this is the interesting thing—I was lying there and I KNEW THIS WAS MY FATHER. I was a baby, a very little baby. I remember that he was wearing a big, big ponytail, and I was surprised. Actually it was a reflection, or a shadow you might say. It was fascinating to me. As it later proved to be—and it later proved to be the case—we saw a picture of him, my parents do have a picture and it looks like he had a ponytail.*

*All right, what I have to say is not going to be a happy letter. Probably, undoubtedly, it will be taken with sadness and grief, but I think that I have — I know what I'm talking about. My English is far from satisfactory, but I do have to say certain things.*

*In my school years, which I will probably keep to a mini-*

mum because I remember all of them and they were interesting to me, but time does go on; anyway my school years
were pretty good years. Apparently as a young child, somewhat after one I would say, I started to do things at a rate
which, uh — showed some of the other people that certain
abilities . . . showed that I was a little bit brighter — at least
a little bit brighter, than other children. I don't want to get
too cocky, or too proud of myself, but that is how I was,
that is how my life started.

Anyway, I started reading, doing things, writing things,
much sooner than a child . . . much sooner. This is unquestionably very much due, in part, to the training that
my mother was giving me. She was and is an extremely
smart woman. Both she and her sister, they are both gifted
in the same way. Both extremely smart women. Also, we
do have a relative in the family who is a very, very intelligent man. I don't think he is quite as smart, but close to it,
and of all the family and relatives we have he is kind of the
third of our — of the three most intelligent. His name is
Babe.

Well, I hope I haven't forgotten what I was saying, because it's hard for me to keep this, to keep my memory
going. Oh, yes, I was as a child—bright. I learned quickly
in school . . . Well, I believe it was second grade, either the
first or second, I skipped half a year and before I was in the
fifth or sixth grade, I skipped another half year. I did finish
sixth grade a year ahead.

We went to Belgium. We left in 1964 — in the beginning of January, and came back to America in 1965. I
started out at the Belgian school, it was a Belgian high
school, I was put back a year so that I was back to my right
age and right school year. I skipped a year and I was put
back a year. Then I went to an English-speaking school and
that's where I was. I really do not have much more to say
about this stuff. It is all explainable and remembered by

my family. They have grand memories of where we were and what we did and I, of course, remember everything that happened.

My problem is, which I want to say right now, is speaking, talking, or whatever you want to call it, I'm talking definitely in the language . . . I'm able to converse, there's no question about that. You see me talking right now, but I'm not really able to keep my thoughts together and my talk straight. I have to use words that— I'm not saying exactly what I mean to say. We went through this before but I'm trying to keep everything going, and I hope that I'm not trying to remember too much.

Life was nice for a young, a young man. I'm not a man, I'm not a child; I'm a young man. We call it that; a person over eighteen is a young man. Shall we say, life for me as a young man was rather beautiful. I— did like life. I liked people and things seemed lovely. Life was nice— I was—

Things went nicely for me as a child. I was able to do things sooner than other children because I was smarter, brighter. I was a quick thinker. I was an adventurer, a trier, these kind of things. I did different things that other children did not do. Of course, a vast percentage of children do do things and their lives are romantic to them. They have kept extremely fond visual memories; well it's the same with myself. It seemed that this boy (speaking of myself) had things going for himself. He was really going to set the world going, glowing. I was going to show the world that I was going to be a success, more than a success; I was going to be someone very well known and admired.

I graduated high school (it's been three years now) and things are very, very different now. It was very nice for the last few years, everything was fine until—pardon the memory, but things were very, very nice until sometime during the eleventh grade. I guess that would be either four or five years ago last March, excuse me, last February, right! —

21

As a young child, I would guess when I was seven or so, I was not feeling well sometimes, these were— My English is horrible! I just don't know what words to use . . . When I was eight years old, sometimes when— I didn't feel well when I went swimming. I would lay down, you know, I would swim and get out of the water, I would lay down and feel kind of dizzy — things were kind of swinging around . . .

We went to see the doctor, I was a child, I didn't know what was going on or anything. They ran tests, it was their problem, it was their concern. I didn't know, it was not my category, or whatever, for me to understand this; I did what I was told, like a child, a youngster. They looked at my head, they gave me an electroencephalogram, which are little electric wire testing devices and other things of that nature. I imagine, I guess now, but I am not sure, that they might have thought I had epilepsy as a child, which apparently I didn't—and don't today. Anyway, they didn't find anything. This may be now, all that I'm saying, this may be all quite inaccurate, because it may very well be as a child I was not told everything. Anyway I was feeling all right all my life. As a matter of fact, I never really thought about that again.

Well, anyway, things were fine; life was beautiful. As a child I did everything and as a teenager I did everything. About a year and a half before I was to graduate high school things were really bad one day. I don't know what day it was, maybe it was a Wednesday. After lunch I just was feeling quite strange, not quite right. I didn't know how to explain it and I didn't know what to do. I just didn't feel good by any means . . . Then there would be these flickerings and perhaps — perhaps I was afraid, perhaps I wasn't, I don't know. I can't say that I remember a hundred per cent correctly. I remember during that day, during that day maybe three times — four times — I had

. . . things would kind of blank out and I would forget things there for a couple of seconds, for two or three seconds and maybe feel a little nauseous and, wow, I was a little bit scared. Of course anyone would be. Not only was it a scary thing to have happen to you, but I was also a child, you know . . . a young teenager perhaps would be more right.

After school I drove home and dropped a couple of friends off, I had a car then. Then when I got home, I got out of the car and I laid down on my bed and I wasn't feeling good. The next thing that apparently happened (my father was sitting down and reading or something, I don't think my mother was there), my father came over and he was shaking me. I was lying on my back and I wasn't feeling well and he was shaking me and shouting, "Josh, Josh, Josh, wake up! Are you all right?" He was shaking me and I had apparently had a breakdown, or convulsion, I don't know what it was, I think something was quite wrong. I did have a convulsion and it went away in about half a minute.

He said, "Calm down, take it easy. I'm going to call the doctor." So they called the doctor and he said go over to the hospital, which was very close, just around the corner from where we lived.

They conducted tests and did try the electroencephalogram, I believe it is called, and talked mostly with my folks. I was not in touch with all of this, but a week later after that, my parents and I went to a hospital — no, not a hospital, we went to see a doctor at a doctor's office, something like that. Anyway it was all explained. They had talked to him and I was told I had epilepsy. It was lucky that I was — some have, some are not curable people, they would have convulsions, there are different types of epilepsy — but mine was of a minor type and with the right drugs things would be OK.

I didn't believe it, I imagine, for maybe six months. I just put it out of my mind. But it really went on and I guess in that little while it was all reality and I took my medicine and everything was fine. I had the right medications, apparently, and it was controllable. I reckoned I could live life.

Well I did, things were forgotten. I mean by forgotten—the hardness, the misery. It's scary and it knocks you down; it depresses you horribly. But after that event, and I don't think it was too long, I got myself back together. I realized I was going to go on and live. As a matter of fact, I don't think anything but that ever occurred to me. I just . . . I probably took it like a young man, you know. It just was OK. It was something new, I had never experienced it before, nobody had, but all right, so I'll go on.

Then things were pretty much OK. It was my final year of high school and I was getting older, I had gotten a car a little while back and I was dating a little bit. I hadn't really zoomed through it, and I hadn't met a million girls yet, but most guys at that age haven't dated at all—real dating or anything. I've done quite a bit, you know, for a guy of my youth.

I was interested in — the way it was — my parents — my mother especially had always told me I was a very, very good-looking young boy, bright, had everything. I mean it was a gift. And it's true, everything she said and told me then was true. I believed her ever since then, and it's been a valuable aid because it's helped me. I've been a strong person, I've understood things, I've been capable and I've been proud of everything. It's very much due to the good work of my mother and father. I actually was the things that I said I am, they were really true. I was smart, good-looking, all of this. This is not . . . if they had never said a thing about this . . . But as it was, it did happen that they saw my capabilities, my abilities, and they helped me and I thank them very much because they have made a good thing out of me. . . .

Actually, I'm quite surprised at this moment, I'm surprised I talked so long about what I have to talk about. At least I've talked a little bit about something; I've talked a little bit about my past and what happened.

I went to college. I went to San Diego State College and things went beautifully. I went through my first year and got almost straight A's. Things went beautifully and after so many years of just being bored with things, junior high and high school and things like that which just didn't interest me—I was going to college and doing extremely well. I'd just go and finish my four years of college and most likely go to law school, attain that and would show the world that I could and would be the greatest. After my first year of college . . . after I finished my first year in college, I'd worked hard all that summer, met more nice young lovelies, and then I went for my second year of college, did very, very well and things were going good in every sense of the word.

Then one year ago last summer, I knew that my parents were moving up north. My mother suggested that she really thought that it was the right thing for me to go, not to go for my next year to a regular college, but to go to a university. That way, after I got out of the university, I'd really have a better than average—a better chance to get to a really fine law school, which makes sense. So we all went up to Santa Barbara except my younger brother, who is doing well in school himself.

One year ago, almost exactly one year ago — We were on a quarter system in that school . . . I went through the first one and things seemed to be going along OK again. We stayed together in that home that we bought. I was in the back room, I was very, very unhappy. Miserable. It was

*very bad, and I was not feeling well. I was sick, just feeling
terrible most of the time and I told the doctor.*

*Well actually, things were going beautifully, one year
ago September when me and my friend Jeff Podemski went
to New York. Everything was a complete one hundred
per cent success. It was incredible, everything that we tried
to do was beyond imagination, all our hitchhiking around
was incredible. We had such luck and it happened so
quickly. Then we met my uncle in New York and he kept—
let us stay at his place for about a week and things were just
great. Then we zoomed back to California and everything
was just great . . . on the trip.*

*Anyway, I had started school and went through the first
quarter. It was just about January now. During that time,
I don't remember exactly when—what weeks or anything—
I was a very, very nervous young man. My hands were always trembling very badly. I was feeling just miserable, my
hands were nervous, I always talked very quickly, as quick
as I could. I always said what I had to say as fast as I
could. That's how it was. I was just nervous, unhappy,
miserable, and just didn't know what to do.*

*I finally did get out of there right at the beginning of
January of this last year, January, 1972, and I finally got an
apartment and I thought maybe things would get better.
But while I was there I was seeing the doctor. He was keeping his eye on me. I was feeling more nervous and sick a
lot of the time. Something was definitely wrong. I didn't
know what was going on.*

*A little less than a year ago, last February, it was Feb-
ruary the 13th — I am — I was in a hospital. One may say,
what's that? I had to go to the hospital — it was a little
strange — my hands were quite, very, you know, nervous.
I was nervous, my whole system was nervous. I was kind of
ruined you might say. I felt bad, everything . . . I was just
not feeling good a-tall, like the cowboy said.*

26

*We went to a doctor, just an* MD. *I told him anything I could tell him about myself and he gave me some stronger medicines but . . . I was still nervous and wasn't feeling too good. Then he said, "I think you better see this other doctor."*

*He was, I believe, a neurosurgeon. I might not have the exact terms, but I know basically what I'm talking about. A surgeon, a brain surgeon—all right, he was kind of, I don't know, for a full doctor, I mean a neurosurgeon, he was kind of (it's hard to say but) he was kind of a giggler, I don't know what age he was, I guess he was around forty-five or fifty — a giggler — you know just a cutie for a doctor — he was hard to imagine you know — laughing. But in his mind he seriously saw that things were wrong and he really didn't tell me, but he told my folks, Mommy and Daddy. My parents were shocked. Could something have happened to Josh? We were all, everybody, we were all a little bit certainly—curious! We didn't know exactly what to do, but we knew that we were going to see the best. You know that this was no joke.*

On Friday morning, February 11, Josh and Leib left for Los Angeles to have a father-son mini-holiday. For two years Josh had been experimenting with filmmaking as a hobby, using a regular 8mm movie camera that we'd bought in 1965 in Europe. It was a very modest piece of equipment and quite inadequate even for an amateur who had moved beyond the home movies stage. They spent a wonderful afternoon camera-hunting in the many Hollywood stores that stock this sort of equipment, and Josh decided on a beautifully compact little Nizo that had most of the capabilities of the more sophisticated products. He decided that he'd buy it when he got out of the hospital. They went to a late afternoon movie, Kubrick's *A Clock-*

*work Orange,* which Josh had seen once before and which had impressed him tremendously in all its aspects—visually, directorially, musically. They ate dinner at one of Hollywood's better old restaurants, Musso & Frank's, and then visited in the evening with Leib's mother, his brother Amnon and Amnon's wife Marilyn. They came home the next day, Saturday, in the early afternoon. Months later Marilyn and Amnon told us how impressed they'd been with Josh's calmness and acceptance, how he'd philosophized about the accidents of nature that select different people for health or illness. He showed reasonable concern but no fear and no self-pity.

Friday morning I had called my parents and my sister, who lived about a hundred miles south of Los Angeles in a retirement community called Sun City, and told them about Josh. I knew they would want to see him as much as he would want to see them. The neurosurgeons, both Dr. Harmon in Santa Barbara and Dr. Stark at UCLA, had been so certain that Josh had a tumor, even before the testing, that try as I might, I could not wish away the knowledge that this would probably be the last time they'd see Josh before he had brain surgery. *Brain surgery!* Oh, the unknown implications of those two words were almost too much to bear. I told them that Josh would be entering the hospital Sunday for a series of tests, but I did not stress my certainty that he did, in fact, have a tumor. Even trying to put it in the most favorable light, I could hear the awful shock and distress in their voices. Worse even than that phone conversation was the one we had later that day with our younger son, Simon. We called him in San Diego and went through the same procedure with him. It was the day before his eighteenth birthday; he was so young, so vulnerable to receive news like that alone and far from home.

On Sunday we arrived at the medical center just before 11 A.M., the hospital check-in time that had been arranged.

Josh, carrying the little suitcase I had packed with his pajamas, robe and a few other things, strode determinedly into that awesome building. We had no way of knowing, or even guessing, that this bright and capable Josh whom we had so loved and enjoyed for twenty years, would never stride back out. Oh, yes, he did leave the hospital five weeks later, but it was a different Josh, with a different kind of beauty and a different wisdom.

We stopped at the admitting desk to sign Josh in. He was expected, the papers were in order and, in keeping with hospital policy, we then had a considerable wait until an aide came for him with a wheelchair. When he was physically able to walk, it was both frustrating and demeaning to Josh to spend so much time waiting to be transported— an experience that was repeated subsequently each time he had to go from one part of the hospital to another. Sometimes the wait lasted almost two hours.

An orderly finally arrived and, with Josh in the wheelchair, we all went to the sixth floor to the two-bed room to which he had been assigned. A young nurse came in and told Josh to get undressed and into bed. We closed the curtain around his bed and stepped out to the corridor for a cigarette while he changed.

When we went back to Josh's room he was in his brightly patterned pajamas, sitting on the side of his bed and talking to the fellow in the next bed. Just about then, lunch was brought around, and while I hung up his clothes and straightened out his nightstand, he ate and chatted with Leib in the best of spirits. After lunch, the pretty young nurse came back and Josh and I answered form questions for about fifteen minutes. We repeated them later when some of the resident physicians came by, and later for several interns. There was a constant bustle of nurses, visitors, interns, television, doctors, food servers, cleaning personnel, aides, and technicians of various sorts; the loudspeaker squawked periodically, summoning doctors or administrators. Someone came by and attached an identifying plastic bracelet to Josh's wrist. A technician came in to take a blood sample. Not all of this activity was centered on Josh, but it flowed all about us; hospitals are not quiet places.

A number of family visitors came—the few who knew of his hospitalization. My parents, his Bubu and Zaida (grandmother and grandfather), had driven up early in the afternoon and spent a little time talking with him. They left soon because of the long drive home. Josh's other grandmother (whose husband had died the previous year) and uncle Amnon came too. By late afternoon things had slowed down and I could tell that Josh was just a little tired from having tried so hard to cheer up all the relatives. It was almost time for the early hospital dinner to be served and Leib and I were worn out and hungry. We were still expecting Simon and we hadn't seen Dr. Stark, although the nurse had told us he would be in to see Josh sometime. We told Josh that we'd go down to the cafeteria on the main floor for a sandwich while he had dinner in his room.

As we emerged from the elevator, we intercepted Simon who had arrived in a state of agitation. His curly mop of hair was disheveled and he was literally jumping with impatience. We embraced him and insisted that he stop with us for a bit to eat before rushing upstairs to Josh. We wanted to calm him down and to clear up some of the questions he started firing at us before we had actually stepped off the elevator. Simon has a persistent way of questioning that is penetrating and obstinate until the last bit of information is forthcoming. It would be much better, I felt, if before he saw Josh we first filled him in on all that we knew. Josh certainly didn't need to be put through that wearing questioning session.

As we sat in the cafeteria explaining to Simon about his

30

brother, I realized that this was the first time we had stopped to review what had happened, and how little we really knew at that point. We told Simon about our visit to Dr. Harmon and our lack of confidence in him. We told about our hurry to reach Dr. Stark, of his eminence in his field, and of the sense of concerned authority he communicated.

"But what about Josh's condition?" he wanted to know.

We told him that both neurosurgeons had conducted preliminary office examinations—testing reflexes, field of vision and eye pressure, and taking down detailed descriptions of Josh's symptoms, which included hand tremors, flickering vision, brief flashes in the brain, momentary losses of memory, general nervousness and malaise. In both cases, the findings had been the same. Josh was suffering some sort of pressure in the left hemisphere of his brain, and all the symptoms indicated the presence of a tumor. The purpose of the tests he would now undergo was to confirm the presence of the suspected growth, to locate it as precisely as possible and to define its extent. There was no way to tell its nature without surgery, and the tests would determine whether surgery was warranted or, for that matter, possible. Dr. Stark had said that although brain surgery is obviously very serious, it is not quite as dangerous as the layman tends to imagine, and there would be every reason to assume that if they did operate Josh would come through very well. There would be some impairment of function, a slight loss of peripheral vision on the right side (which Josh already felt) and a temporary difficulty with speech patterns. On the basis of the description of the symptoms, the amount of pressure and other factors, all possible speed was indicated. Brain tumors grow erratically and, at certain points in their development, very rapidly. The educated guess of both surgeons had been that without treatment Josh had perhaps six months to live.

"No," Leib said in response to Simon's question, "they don't know what causes these tumors. But probably what was diagnosed a few years ago as an epileptic seizure wasn't that at all but some early manifestation of a growth." The medication that Josh had been taking to control the probably nonexistent epilepsy had in fact been disguising the fact that he had a growth in his brain.

That was all we knew. It was a serious thing, but there seemed to be every reason to be quite hopeful about the outcome.

It had been a good idea, stopping first to talk to Simon. He was more relaxed and calm by the time we returned to Josh's room together. And, for ourselves, it had been helpful just to stop for a moment to review the situation. Perhaps it really wasn't so grim. It was a shocker all right but there was a lot to hope for, and the alternative, six months to live, was too unreal to be believed. Josh was very cheerful when we got to his room and was delighted to see Simon. They started talking and laughing and having a great brotherly visit. While we'd been downstairs, Dr. Stark had stopped in briefly but, Josh told us, hadn't had anything new to say, just that tests of various sorts would start the next day.

We must have stayed until eight-thirty or nine o'clock. It had been a very long day and we still had the ride back to Santa Barbara ahead of us, while Simon had to nurse his jalopy back to San Diego. When we left, Josh was in good spirits, planning to watch television until he fell asleep for the night. We promised to be back the following day in the early afternoon. I kissed Josh good-night, Leib and Simon shook hands with him, and we left.

On the way back to Santa Barbara, Leib and I speculated about the tests, what would show up, what the next step would be. I felt absolutely certain, because the doctors' diagnoses had been so similar, that the tests would confirm the presence of a tumor. Nor had Dr. Stark indicated any other possible explanation for the symptoms, which I felt sure he would have done if there had been any doubt in his mind as to what the problem was. I had gotten the impression somehow, more from his facial expression than from his exact words, that there was no doubt of the necessity for surgery—only whether or not the growth would be operable.

Leib disagreed. He felt that there was a very good chance that an operation would not be necessary, that perhaps some other, less serious reason for the pressure would be found. Almost in tears, he said, "Oh, I hope he won't have to be operated on!"

I remember replying, "I hope that it is operable. If it isn't, that'll be a death sentence."

For reasons very different from those we each had in mind during that conversation, he proved to be so right, and I was so wrong.

The next day, Monday, Josh wasn't in his room when we arrived, and the fellow in the next bed told us that he was out having some tests. We chatted with him a bit and soon Josh was brought back in a wheelchair by an orderly. He was in very good spirits and very hungry. Leib went to the cafeteria and brought up a hamburger and a malted which Josh ate while he told us about the various tests he'd had so far. There had been an extensive series of X rays taken of his head, another electroencephalogram, more blood samples and urine samples. He was still scheduled to take brain scans, the angiogram, and he didn't know what else. It was a colossal bore waiting to be wheeled around, but so far nothing they had done had been physically painful.

"Some of the nurses are real cute," he informed us, "but the staff doctors and the interns are a drag. Troops of them come clumping through, morning and night, and I feel like a monkey in the zoo."

One of the nurses had told him that his doctor, Dr. Stark, was the man who had operated on a television star, an operation that had been much in the news because of the young woman's popularity, and now Josh felt quite assured that we really had the top man working on him. He thought most of the nonmedical personnel—the orderlies, the cleanup crew, the fellows who pushed the wheelchairs around—were very nice. The X-ray technicians were cruddy, though—very impressed with their own importance. Not so bad in the other departments he'd been to. It was a real Josh outpouring. He was observing everything, everyone. He was interested in the workings of the hospital and already knew most of the people by name.

While he was eating dinner, two of the residents came through with a group of perhaps eight or ten interns and students. The doctors acknowledged our existence with nods and mumbled greetings of some sort. The others stood mute in a cluster at the foot of the bed. One of the doctors took the chart, asked Josh how he was feeling, and then, turning to the group of acolytes, described Josh in medical terminology. Then they herded themselves out of the room. I could see them moving down the hall and into another room. Josh made a vulgar gesture at their backs as they left, then turned to me and we burst out laughing. This parade, which had been quite unpleasant, though for no immediately definable reason, occurred several times each day.

Dr. Stark stopped in at about eight o'clock for a few minutes. He told us, "I can't give you any more information until the tests are all completed and we've had a chance to study the results, but by Wednesday evening or Thursday at the latest, we'll know just where we stand."

Tentatively, however, he was scheduling the surgery for Friday, keeping his calendar free and arranging for the operating theater. He talked for a few more minutes with

Josh, wanted to know if he was getting along all right, and then he left. I was watching Josh to see how he reacted to the doctor's words. He seemed calm enough. I couldn't see any fear on his face. 1824667

After the doctor left, Josh looked at us. I suppose we looked terribly grim, and he smiled. "Come on. You knew what we had to expect. You don't think a neurosurgeon is going to let a great brain like mine get away, do you?"

The next day we didn't arrive at the hospital until late afternoon. Leib had considerable work to do at the office, and several customers had to be rescheduled since it was apparent that he would not be able to work for at least a week. With the huge medical problem we had facing us, we had to maintain our business contacts, who constituted our only source of income. Besides, Josh would be involved in tests and we probably wouldn't be able to see him until late afternoon anyway. We stopped in Westwood and I got Josh some more pajamas. When we got to Josh's room, he was lying in bed with his eyes closed, rather pale. He wasn't asleep, because as soon as we came in he opened his eyes and looked at us with such intense anger and hostility that it was quite alarming. Before we could do more than say hello, before we could even ask how he was feeling or what was wrong, it all came spewing forth in a flood. That afternoon he had had the angiogram. It was sheer horror. They had inserted tubes in the veins of his groin and he could feel them being pushed through his body. The procedure had taken what seemed hours to him. His body felt violated, his person abused. And then they had injected the dye. His brain had felt as though it was going to burst. There had been an indescribably horrible pain behind his eyes, as though daggers were being pushed through his eyeballs from the back. And heat—intense heat. His brain and eyes felt seared. The more he talked, the more his anger lessened. He had had to give vent to his fear and pain and frustration to somebody.

There wasn't much we could say. We were sorry, more sorry than we could tell him, but it was a procedure that had to be performed. Had it lasted long? The actual searing pain had been short. Well, couldn't he just put it aside, put it out of his mind? It was too horrible! The worst thing about it was that they hadn't warned him—they hadn't told him what to expect. They were treating him like a guinea pig.

By the time his dinner arrived Josh was feeling much better, but the first seed of distrust of the doctors, of the whole medical setup had been planted. It could have been so easily avoided had they just explained to him what to expect.

*We headed to someone who apparently is the finest at UCLA. There are a few different men in all of the country, from side to side, perhaps five or six or seven or eight, who knows, ten—you know, different surgeons who vary slightly about what is needed to be done when it comes to brain tumors. Because that's what we were worried about, that I might be having a tumor growing in my brain. And it so happened, I'll tell you right away, yes, we found that out.*

*Now I guess that it was in February, in February, 1972, I think it was, I don't know, the 9th or 10th, somewhere I guess about there. Anyway, we talked to Dr. Stark. He had just operated on, I guess her name was [a well-known TV actress], a few weeks before that. She had needed a brain operation and I had heard of them before over the years, but it sounded awfully scary. I was so proud (I don't know if that's the correct word)—it was so fine to hear a young woman to be so brave—to know what may happen to her,* to have an operation on her head. Anyway, the doctor's name is Dr. Stark. I also wound up having him as my operator.

We didn't know what would be the eventual end but we did know we would have to go to the hospital to have tests taken on me, so I remember the date. It was the same year and day I mentioned, it was February, February the— We went around Hollywood looking at what was going on, and I bought myself a camera. I was looking around because I had wanted to become, perhaps on the sidelines, a film-maker. I felt I had a certain amount of ambition and ability and I could really . . . I remember February 12th, and then there was February 13th. It was on a Sunday and that was the day they took me to a room in the hospital.

I — what did I do? I just lay back and they took all kinds of tests on me Monday, Tuesday and Wednesday. Tests all day, all day from early in the morning, I think something like eight in the morning to late in the evening— just taking tests . . . just taking tests.

One of them was just a horrible test. It's the angiogram, and what they did in that one . . . it was a horrible experience and — I'm not kidding, it was the worst thing that's ever happened to me in my life. I say this—I wouldn't go through that thing again. It was unbelievable. My system was not in good condition—you know for the past couple of months I had not been feeling good.

I had to lay down and they had to— when they had to clean me off, should I say, and give me shots but the main thing, you know, was they take a long tube — I don't know what the correct term was, I don't know what it was — a plastic tube, no that's not the right thing, let's see, a tube, let's say a quarter inch, a quarter inch thick — a long tube like a— oh boy . . .

I really can't think of anything . . . Things aren't going so hot with my memory.

37

*Anyway, I was told I had to lie down, and there were a couple of people around me. I'll say this, I couldn't stand the people that were there. There was this man and his job was—well, he would be doing the work. There were two women, a black woman and a Mexican; they made me sick. They were really annoying, you know. I mean they weren't really deliberately going out to cut me, but when you're nervous, and my head wasn't feeling good, everything wasn't feeling well, you know. I mean, there was a stupid little woman with her stupid little friend. They'd giggle and they'd tickle me. They weren't talking to me; they were just giggling at one another and it was very annoying.*

*They cut me open down the middle of the stomach and they put this long plastic tube all the way from the middle of my groin—all the way up. It's underneath — it's inside my stomach — you couldn't see it. They would stick it up — They were pushing it up all the way up, up, up, up and there—it's in the middle of my neck, and then they were sticking it all the way up into the middle of my head. Now, it's in my head, there's a tube there, and they stick it somewhere in my head, I don't know exactly where, near the middle, near the side. It's like a long plastic tube, like an air tube or something, and it's in my head, all inside my body. And then they were doing all these electrical tests; I don't know anything about them but they were painful beyond belief. It was unbelievable!!*

*I'm stopping right here. I won't discuss any more about that — but it was terrible. So they were doing all kinds of tests on me for the full three days. It was on a Monday and a Tuesday and a Wednesday.*

*Wednesday night Dr. Stark said he was pretty sure that, well, more than pretty sure, that there was a real tumor there growing away in my head and it had to be operated on. I was kind of unhappy. I was in a terrible state of mind . . . I just felt terrible I was having— I always get off the*

*track! OK, let's say Monday they did some testing, Tues-*
*day they did some testing — Wednesday I got the bad*
*news, that Wednesday night, that they would have to*
*operate on me — they would do it Friday.*

We rushed back on Wednesday in fear of what we might find after the unfortunate occurrences of the previous day with the angiogram. We arrived just after lunchtime. Josh was reading and motioned us to be quiet when we came in. The man in the other bed had just been brought back from surgery. He was heavily sedated, and numerous tubes attached to various parts of his body emerged from under the sheet. Periodically he groaned. We spoke for a few minutes with his wife, whom we'd seen several times before, and she told us that he'd come through the operation just fine and that there had been no malignancy. Good news. Josh told us that he had no further tests scheduled for that afternoon, so we all decided to go downstairs to the cafeteria for some coffee where we could talk more freely without disturbing the other patient, and for a change of scenery for Josh.

Over coffee Josh told us that he'd had the brain scans. The only difference between that and X rays is that he had to keep his head still in various positions for five to ten minutes at a time, but, aside from being a nuisance, it didn't hurt. So far as he knew, there were no more tests scheduled. Dr. Stark would be in later, about six, and wanted to speak with all of us then.

Josh had been giving much thought to the upcoming surgery he would probably be having and had decided that he really didn't want to wait to get that camera he had selected. Would we go to Hollywood tomorrow and get it for him before we came to the hospital? He had his checkbook with him in his room and he had made out a check to us for two hundred dollars. We said we'd get it for him and to forget the check, but he was very insistent that he pay for it.

He talked about the other man in the room and about how happy he was that the trouble with his yarbles (a word from *A Clockwork Orange*) would be okay. "After all," he said, "next to a brain, they're one's most important part."

Simon came up again late in the afternoon. We took him out to dinner at a restaurant in Westwood. He just couldn't seem to grasp that this was happening to Josh. We told him that everything seemed to indicate Josh would be undergoing an operation and that, indeed, surgery was tentatively scheduled for Friday. We went back to Josh's room for a while and Josh told Simon all about the angiogram. He tried to make this account more amusing than awful, but I think Simon got some of the picture of what it was like. Simon left shortly after that—there was the long ride back to San Diego.

Josh and I were playing Go Fish with a deck of cards I'd bought for him when Dr. Stark came in. The doctor was very interested to know how the game was going—how Josh was doing. I realized that he was trying to establish what degree of mental dysfunction Josh was suffering, but, in fact, Josh's memory was perfect, as usual. He was soundly defeating me.

Dr. Stark said, "There is no question now as to the necessity for the operation. Josh has a tumor in the left hemisphere of his brain, it is very deeply placed, almost in the center of the brain, but just to the left. All the indications are that it can be favorably excised, but we'll have more details tomorrow when we've had more time to analyze all of the information from the tests."

Josh wanted a description of the surgical techniques that would be used. What exactly would they do to his head?

Dr. Stark drew a rough sketch and showed us how an incision would be made circling up from the front of the left ear to the top of the head and then back down the center for about four inches. This flap of skin would be folded back, four holes would be drilled through the skull and then the exposed rectangle of bone would be sawed loose, removed, and set aside until the surgery was completed. After the tumor had been removed and the operation was over, the bone would be replaced and secured with wires, the skin flap would be sewn into place, and the procedure would be concluded. He assured Josh that there would be actually very little disfigurement. Of course there would be a very long scar, but it would be no more than a hairline thick and, once his hair had grown in, it would be virtually invisible.

What else should Josh be prepared to face? Well, there wouldn't be too much pain—more discomfort than actual pain. He would have a little temporary memory distortion and some difficulty with his speech. There would be a permanent loss of some peripheral vision in his right eye. After he recuperated, the only limitation on his physical activities would be to avoid any contact sports. He would still be maintained on anticonvulsion drugs for a period of time, because the internal scar tissue of the surgery might—just might—create some problems, but that was something to be dealt with later. When could he plan to return to school? Well, perhaps it would be best to aim for the fall quarter in September; better not to think in terms of the summer session.

When the doctor had left, all of us felt better because at least we knew exactly what to expect. It was bad, but not intolerable. And once Josh had recovered, everything would be just fine, just as good as it had ever been. We left Josh in a very good mood and drove home feeling quite confident that things were going favorably.

Thursday morning we left early again, since we first had to go to Hollywood to get the camera for Josh. We bought it and added, as an extra little gift, some lens attachments and several rolls of film. Then we had a quick lunch and went to the hospital. Josh was ecstatic over the camera. He quickly read the instruction manual and kept focusing and adjusting and jiggling knobs. It was even better than he remembered. He couldn't wait to get out of the hospital to start filming.

"Boy, it's going to be fabulous! All that time before I have to go back to school! I'll make movies that will make history!"

That afternoon there was an even more steady stream of doctors and interns than there had been on other days. The neurosurgery residents, some of whom would be assisting during surgery, all assured us that Dr. Stark was the best and that everything would be fine. Another doctor, the anesthesiologist, came up to examine Josh. The whole atmosphere around Josh that day seemed so positive.

Some of the family came by again early in the evening, including his cousin Fabe. Josh wanted to know if we'd contacted his friends Jeff and Larry in San Diego. We told him that we had and that they'd probably be up to see him over the weekend. He was a little disappointed that he wouldn't see them before the operation, but they had school and part-time jobs and it was tough to get away.

Dr. Stark was there again at about seven. He was smiling! The tests had been very encouraging. Josh's tumor was encapsulated (contained in a discrete mass), and the surgery should go well. Josh would be shaved and prepped at about six o'clock the next morning. Surgery would probably start about seven. "It's a complex procedure," he said, "so don't expect it to be over before two or three in the afternoon."

We said, "We'll be here at six."

Josh protested adamantly that he did not want us to come. He said there was no need. He wasn't anxious for us to see him get his head shaved, and that's all we would see. We'd just have to sit around and worry for too many hours. Dr. Stark didn't disagree. There was really nothing we could do to help, and it would be more beneficial if we could get a good night's rest so that we'd be better able to help Josh through the period after the operation. Two o'clock was absolutely the earliest we'd need to come to the hospital. So that was decided.

Before leaving, Dr. Stark emptied the things from his pockets and asked Josh to match them with little slips of paper on which words were written—knife with knife, wallet with wallet, keys with keys, and so on. Josh did it with no hesitation or difficulty. Again, no evidence of malfunctioning in his communications processes. Dr. Stark bade us good-night and left.

I don't know how late we stayed with Josh. Certainly it was past ten when we left. We had talked quietly through the evening. We all felt that Josh was fortunate to have Dr. Stark as his doctor. He would do the very best job, no question of that. Shortly before we left, Josh said, "I'm sorry that I turned out to be such a son. What a disappointment I must be to you. A guy with a ruined brain."

We did what we could to assure him that that was the farthest thing from our minds, that we were incredibly proud of him, his courage, his manliness. We told him how much we loved him, what a truly wonderful person we thought he was. His brain was not ruined, he was not ruined. Everything was going to be fine. We really meant it. We really believed that to be true. I think Josh almost believed it, too.

February 18, 1972. Our son was in surgery in UCLA Medical Center while we were in Santa Barbara trying to control our impatience, our desire to be with him, our fears, and our apprehension. We simply could not wait until two o'clock, although we had promised not to come before then. We must have arrived at the hospital at about noon. We went to the sixth floor and the nurse told us that there had been no word from surgery; we hadn't expected that there would be. She directed us to a waiting room down one of the corridors and told us that we would be notified as soon as there was any information concerning Josh.

We sat down and waited. Time stood still. I was constantly aware during all of this waiting period that Josh was in mortal danger, but the situation was too threatening, too overwhelming, too catastrophic to be truly comprehended. I just recall sitting there and feeling that things would have to be all right because they couldn't be otherwise. Josh was too young, too strong, too capable, too promising, too beautiful for anything to go wrong. Dr. Stark was the best there was. This hospital had the finest facilities available. Surely—surely, things would be all right.

Two o'clock . . . three o'clock. We walked back to the nurse's desk. No word from surgery yet. Leib went downstairs and brought up coffee for us. Four o'clock. Our feelings of apprehension began to increase; the sense of impending disaster, the terrible fear that something may have conceivably gone wrong. They had been down there so long. Something awful was delaying them.

It was impossible to sit still any longer. I stood in the hallway, walked back and forth up the corridor toward the nurse's desk, toward the elevator, back down to the waiting room, back and forth.

Leib came to join me in the corridor. From where we stood in the hallway, we could see through the waiting room windows that overlooked the city. It was dark now. The sun had set.

Suddenly we saw Dr. Stark walking down the corridor

44

toward us. There was something ominous in his manner, his bearing. The erect posture and the confident look that he wore on all the other occasions we had seen him were gone. There was an appearance of defeat about him; perhaps there was anger, too. I thought to myself, "He's exhausted." I glanced at my watch and saw it was past six-thirty. The operation had been in progress for almost twelve hours.

As he came toward us, we rushed down the corridor to meet him. Both of us quickly asked, "Is Josh all right? Is he alive?"

He said, "Yes, Josh is alive. He's in the recovery room now and he will be brought up soon, but I must speak with you first."

He motioned us into a room off the corridor. It was a small classroom; the sign on the door indicated that it was a nurse's lecture room. We went in with the doctor and took seats in front of the desk. Behind the doctor, as we sat looking at him, was a blackboard. It was as though we were schoolchildren about to get a lecture from the teacher. The lesson turned out to be one that would change the entire pattern of our lives.

The doctor sat still for a moment, looked at us, and then said, "The operation was not as successful as I had hoped. The tumor was not benign. Your son has a malignant growth in his brain. I was not able to remove all of it; I got as much as I could." At that point, his face flushed red and tears came to his eyes.

I realize now that, in a sense, he was almost more upset than we at that particular moment because he was able to anticipate what we would have to live through—what our son would have to suffer before his death. We had no way of knowing what lay ahead. We had no way of foreseeing the difficulties, the degree of discomfort, the misery that Josh would suffer.

We had so many questions to ask the doctor, but we were so shocked, so frightened, there was no place to start. I have a vivid mental image of his standing up and turning to the blackboard and writing across it. I can see that word in front of my mind's eye, ASTROCYTOMA. "That is what I think it is that your son has. However, there will have to be a more extensive biopsy before we determine the exact nature of the tumor; but I am absolutely certain that is what it is. The tests will indicate the more specific character of the tumor and will help in determining any further treatment."

He sat down heavily and said, "The tumor was not removable in its entirety because it was not encapsulated. It was not easy to reach and it was—" and at that he stopped, put his hands together, and locked together his fingers. "That is the way the tumor was, it was entwined in the brain. If I had cut out any more than I did remove, I would have done such extensive damage to Josh that he would not have been able to function at all."

Oh, it was unbelievable. We asked him what would happen now, what we had to anticipate, what Josh had to anticipate. He told us that Josh should recover quite well from the surgery. He would have some good time before a decline finally set in. In the interim there were various treatments that could be attempted; the first one, as soon as his recovery from surgery would permit, would be to start cobalt radiation to try to inhibit further growth of the tumor that remained. After that, we would see what else might be done. Josh would be needing continuing medical attention. There was no way to predict the exact course of the illness but, to the best of his knowledge, the tumor that Josh had was an incurable malignancy.

We asked one more question. "How long does Josh have?"

He said he could not answer it, that there was no way to

46

tell, but—and again his face flushed red and there were tears in his eyes—"Count months, not years."

This short meeting with Dr. Stark could not have taken more than ten or fifteen minutes. We were really in too deep a state of shock to ask all the appropriate questions, to elicit a great deal of information. At the same time, Dr. Stark was totally exhausted from the grueling day he had spent in surgery and from the awful knowledge that he had operated unsuccessfuly—that is, the tumor he had hoped to be able to excise was both malignant and not entirely removable, and was, in effect, a death sentence for his patient.

There was nothing more to say then. We just wanted to see our son. Dr. Stark thought Josh would be up from the recovery room by this time and walked with us down the hall and down another corridor to the Intensive Care Unit. Josh was lying in bed—very still, pale, quiet. We hadn't seen him that morning—at his request, of course—when they had shaved his head, and now all we could see was a large bandage completely covering his head and distorting its shape. There was no way really to tell what he looked like without it. His face was somewhat pale but not alarmingly so, and there was a slight discoloration around his left eye. He was lying on his right side, the left side of his head being the portion that had been operated on. The doctor came in with us and stood on one side of the bed, at Josh's back, as we walked around to the side where he could see us.

I took Josh's hand and we looked down at him and smiled. He was conscious. He looked at us, tried to smile back at us. He was very weak, very tired, but alert and completely cognizant of our being there. I looked at him and said, "Joshie, Joshie, how are you, sweetheart? How is everything?"

He looked very carefully back at me. It was a long look

47

and there was just the hint of a rueful smile at the corner of his lips. He didn't answer, but the hand I was holding moved from mine and he made that most common of young male gestures, the closed fist with the extended middle finger.

In that one gesture he had succinctly analyzed, accepted, and defied the reality of the situation that existed. It was so perfect a gesture, so perfect a summation of the situation, that it dissipated the awful tension of that hideous day. Both of us had to laugh. Even Dr. Stark had a smile on his face. With that, the doctor motioned us to leave and Josh closed his eye, the one that we could see, and we left the room.

*Friday they did the operating. It was a long operation. It took, let me get my bearings straight now, somewhere in the neighborhood of, and it's not wild imagination, but either nine and a half hours or ten and a half hours. It was a long, long thing and it wasn't — they found out afterwards, that they couldn't — they saw the tumor there but they couldn't cut it all out. It was right in the center. It was deep as possible, as centralized as possible. They could cut some, Dr. Stark and the other surgeons, but if they would have cut any more they would have made a vegetable out of me. I would have been living, I imagine, but I would have been a fruitless vegetable. What kind of life is that? It's just a nothingness.*

*Then I was taken over to Intensive Care, all wrapped up with a big blanket on my head. They sewed my head together with electric wires—electric is not the correct word, they were metal wires to hold it together, things like that, and I was in Intensive Care for a while. I'm not going to talk about all that, all the minutes and hours and days that I spent.*

48

*I was in the hospital for an exact five weeks. A full five weeks. It was like an eternity. It felt like years—there was just no way to compare it. I guess now things are getting a little straightened out in my mind and things are believable. You don't know time — it goes on and on. Thinking, thinking they just mixed up my mind and goofed up my head and all those other explanations. Time was just hard to believe anyway.*

We left the hospital silently. Neither of us seemed able to say anything. We had to have some time, individually, to comprehend what we had been told, to grasp the full implications of a malignant brain tumor that was killing Josh. It was late in the evening, very cold. We were quite numb with exhaustion.

For the first part of our trip back to Santa Barbara, we didn't speak. After we had driven about halfway back, Leib looked at me, quickly as he was driving, and in the most agonized tone of voice said, "What did we do wrong? What have we done wrong?"

I had already asked myself that question and I had absolutely rejected it as having no validity. We had done nothing wrong. We had tried ever since Josh's birth to be good, concerned parents. I don't mean to imply that we never made any mistakes, but certainly they were not so gross as to lead to a catastrophe of this sort. We had always maintained close medical supervision over him; we never neglected any of his ailments. I felt that if we didn't at this moment expunge all sense of personal guilt, we would be unable to function in Josh's best interests. We would have to work with, and live with, and try to accommodate ourselves to Josh's medical and emotional needs from now on. Guilt, needlessly self-imposed, would have incapacitated us, making us incapable of helping our son.

49

I turned to Leib and said rather harshly, "Stop it! Stop it immediately. We are not guilty, we have done nothing wrong. This is an accident of nature. This is a horror, a random horror, but we are not responsible for it happening and we must not permit that thought to cloud our future, whatever that future might hold."

Then we begin discussing the problem in terms of the immediate future. Certain things were quite obvious, however shocking to us, from our talk with Dr. Stark. Josh was suffering from a malignancy, a brain cancer. There was no known medical cure for it at this time. However, there were some further techniques that could be used for his treatment. First among them, as soon as his recovery from surgery would permit, would be a five- or six-week treatment with cobalt therapy. After that, the doctor indicated, Josh would have to be under continuing medical care and observation. We could not project, nor could he project, further into the future than that.

Immediately, we were faced with the obvious problem of the distance between our home in Santa Barbara and the UCLA medical facility where he was now, and where he would continue to be treated under the supervision of the doctor who, we hoped, would remain in charge of his case. We would have to arrange to be closer to UCLA so as to have Josh closer to its facilities.

We had both been thinking along the same lines. First, we considered the possibility of my renting a furnished apartment in the area of UCLA, with Leib coming down whenever possible. When Josh was discharged from the hospital, he and I would be close to the facility during his cobalt therapy. After that, we would see what the future required.

On the other hand, we had been just a short time in Santa Barbara. Although I was happy there and had hoped it would be our permanent home, Leib had never been as comfortable there as I was. He missed Los Angeles, the feeling of a "big city." With this new terror hanging over us and this new requirement to be nearer UCLA, perhaps there wasn't enough to keep us in Santa Barbara. It was true that we had invested a half year of our time working hard to get a toehold in the real-estate business, but we certainly hadn't established ourselves that well, nor had we so much at stake to prevent us from giving it up, not as a bad job but, under pressure of circumstances, as a move that had not proved to be practical. We could return to the Los Angeles area and, although it would mean more financial setbacks and a little further delay, Leib felt sure he could re-establish himself in another real-estate office.

There were, in addition, some other considerations. We were newcomers in Santa Barbara. I had only one old friend there. We had made some new acquaintances, some of them very pleasant, but we certainly had no long-term attachments. Josh hadn't really had time to make friends there; he had just begun to make a few social contacts. If we returned to Los Angeles, Josh would be able to see the young people he knew well. What family we had in California were either based in the Los Angeles area or lived further south and were therefore closer to Los Angeles than to Santa Barbara. The arguments in favor of another move were strong.

When we got home, we again had to make that series of dreadful phone calls. I called my parents and told them the results of the operation. I spoke with Simon and again tried to help him, from a distance, to accept and not be too frightened or too negative about what we could project for the future. Leib spoke with his mother and his brother. It was awful, it was just awful. With each repetition we were ourselves beginning to absorb it all. Each time we came closer to the realization and acceptance of the fact that Dr. Stark told us our son was terminally ill with cancer of the brain.

Leib is fortunate in that, regardless of circumstances, regardless of problems or worries, he can usually sleep. Indeed, later that night when we finally retired, after we had gone over and reconsidered all the options open to us, all the possibilities for assisting our son, for accommodating his future needs, he was able to fall asleep.

I am, and always have been, an insomniac. Once I was in bed, I thought about what I was really hoping for my son. I adored that child, I loved that boy so much. My firstborn, my wonderful Josh. But as much as I wanted him to live, as much as I wanted to believe that some miracle would occur, that we would be able to find some new approach, some happy resolution to what faced him, another portion of me was screaming in my mind, "Let him die tonight, let him die tonight. He doesn't know what's happening, he's not suffering now. Must he go through what lies ahead?"

I answered myself, "How could you think that? That's inhuman, that's unnatural, that's unmotherly. Surely you want your boy to live."

And I replied to myself, "Of course I want my son to live, but I want him to have a life that's worth living. If all he can look forward to is a horrible deterioration, pain and a slow death, that can't be good. He would be better off dead, now."

Then my conventional sense of reason again came to the fore and said, "No, no, that's not true. Even though the operation was not a success, the cobalt will work and if that doesn't work, somewhere in this world there is some other treatment that is going to work. Josh is not only going to recover, he is going to be exactly as he was before. He is going to live a long, full life. He is going to be well, he is going to be productive, he is going to accomplish all that he wanted. The other is impossible, it is unacceptable, it cannot be. Josh is not dying, he will recover."

Early the next morning, during that seemingly endless hundred-mile journey back to the UCLA hospital, we again discussed the possibility of moving back to the Los Angeles area. All things considered—the availability of medical help, our familiarity with the area, the proximity of friends and relatives, and Leib's certainty that he could re-establish himself there in a short period of time—we decided it was the best thing to do. The distance from Santa Barbara to Los Angeles was too great to maintain Josh's treatment from our present home. Leib and I would need each other's support during this time and it would be financially more burdensome for us to have to maintain two homes. A home base in Santa Barbara was untenable. We would move.

Our first concern, however, was to see our son. We got to the hospital early in the morning and saw him again briefly in the Intensive Care Unit. He recognized us, I'm sure, but he was unable to speak. We spoke to him, as the doctor had instructed us to, quietly, slowly, one at a time. We saw that he had difficulty comprehending what we were saying, but that was to be expected so soon after brain surgery. We did not stay long; we were not permitted to.

Later Dr. Stark came and spoke to us for a moment. He told us that he would be away for the coming week and was turning over the immediate care of Josh to his colleague Dr. Crawford, another of the senior neurosurgeons at the UCLA facility. He assured us that Josh would be in capable hands. Everything at this time seemed to be basically under control. Nothing unusual had occurred during the night and he felt that things were going along as well as could be expected.

We had told all the relatives that it would be absolutely inappropriate for them to come to the hospital Saturday to see Josh. It was too soon after the operation. They were concerned, we knew, but we suggested that they should not come before Sunday, at the very earliest. Therefore, Saturday for Josh was a quiet day. We saw him for brief moments a few times that morning. Then we went out and started to look for an apartment in the area.

I had always disliked the heat and the smog of Los Angeles, as did Josh. Leib and I decided, in view of UCLA's location in Westwood, about five or six miles from the beach, to try to get an apartment in the nearby Santa Monica area as it would be cooler in summer and less smoggy.

We made another decision. Josh was an intelligent and sensitive young man. He knew that we had taken a big gamble in moving up to Santa Barbara. If he was made to feel entirely responsible for our return to the Los Angeles area, he would feel guilty for imposing tremendous burdens on us. We decided to present the new move to him truthfully, but in the best possible light. Josh should in no way feel that his illness had precipitated a move that made us unhappy. Quite the contrary, we felt very positive about it. These were two important decisions: to be honest with Josh, no matter what the future held, and to put everything in the most positive manner possible.

We scoured the Santa Monica area looking for apartments. This was a new experience for us as we are not apartment dwellers. We rapidly found that the only apartments that would create an environment of comfort, a degree of privacy, and a feeling of, if not affluence, at least not the opposite, would be extremely expensive. Finally we selected three possibilities ranging upward in price from exorbitant to outrageous. We decided to choose one the following day when Simon came up; we wanted him to help us make the decision since his response to the apartments was likely to be closer to Josh's.

We saw Josh intermittently during the day, perhaps half a dozen times. There was no appreciable change. He was very quiet, and he was awake on and off for a few moments each time we saw him. We spoke to him slowly, carefully; we smiled, we were as cheerful as we could be. I think we did a good job in that. There were no tears, no weeping. I don't think we communicated any sense of disaster.

It was a very strange day. On the one hand, filled with determination and decision, we were busy making complex plans for the future that would redirect most of our activities. On the other hand, we were in a sort of limbo. Josh had such a strange quality to him, such a vague, lost, unresponsive look when we spoke to him. It was difficult when we were with him to believe that we were in the real world, that this nightmare was actually happening.

Sunday morning, before we came down to UCLA again, we started making more specific arrangements for the move that we had decided upon. Leib went to the office for a short time to talk to the broker for whom we worked and explain to him our decision to leave. I notified Josh's roommate in Isla Vista of the outcome of Josh's surgery, that it was definite Josh would not be returning, that we would all be moving. I asked him if he would get Josh's things together so that we could pick them up before our move. I don't remember all the other things we took care of that morning. I do remember that, being in the business, we had "For Sale" signs in the garage and we put one on the front lawn of our home. Then we left for UCLA.

When we arrived around noon, my parents were there. Gradually, as the day wore on, Josh's uncle Ben-Ami arrived from New York, then Amnon and Marilyn, then my mother-in-law. In the corridor and in the waiting room down the hall there was a profusion of people, but not around Josh; that was carefully controlled. Besides us, only his grandparents were permitted to see him individually, for a moment. We were bombarded with questions from relatives and found ourselves having to repeat to each of them in turn the information we had, particularly with regard to what we could expect for Josh's future.

Josh seemed to me to be somewhat better. He appeared to be a little more alert and he did try to speak; not much, a couple of words, but they made sense and were in response to specific questions. He had no pain. As far as his appearance went, his color was reasonably good. The left eye was starting to discolor rapidly, for he had sustained tremendous shocks to the left portion of his skull and it was logical that his left eye should blacken. There was, as well, a small red blood clot on the eyeball itself. Outside of that, however, his appearance was not distressing and he was kept quite comfortable in the Intensive Care Unit and dozed intermittently.

I believe that afternoon Josh's good friends, Jeff and Larry, came up from San Diego. I really don't remember. I do know many people came and went during the day. Most of them weren't permitted to see Josh but they wanted to be close, to offer moral support.

Simon arrived at about three. After he saw Josh for a few moments, we left with him to show him the apartments we had tentatively selected and explained our decision to return to Los Angeles. With his help, we picked a pleasant, third-floor apartment designed so that it did not look out upon another building. From the front wall of glass, which opened on to a balcony, there was a lovely view of the hills in the distance and, nearer, of palm trees. It was a quiet building, and we shared a common wall with only one other apartment, so there would be adequate privacy for Josh. In addition to Josh's bedroom and ours, there was a den that Simon could occupy during the summer. Although it was extremely expensive, we felt that in terms of Josh's comfort the money would be as well spent as any medical costs we would be incurring.

As we drove back to the hospital with Simon, we told him everything the doctor had told us, trying to be as precise as possible and yet to present it in a way that would be tolerable. Simon looked at us with tears and said, "Oh, I have had for the last few days such a terrible pain in my heart, such a pain in my heart." There was very little that we could do to relieve that pain. He was struggling, as we were, to accept this horror that had befallen Josh.

Back at the hospital, late in the afternoon, we suggested to the relatives who were still there that it really would be best if they left. Gradually, by ones and twos, the place emptied. We saw Josh once more. It wasn't late but there was no purpose in our staying any longer either. We were getting terribly tired and we had so much to do. We said good-night to Josh and left.

The next few days were very busy. There were dozens of things to attend to. Looking back on it now, I wonder how we managed to get everything done in such an efficient manner when our thoughts were so much on Josh. We arranged for a moving company, sold our house and some furnishings, picked up Josh's things and brought his car to the apartment, turned unfinished escrows over to our broker, transferred our checking account and did whatever else was necessary for the move, while still visiting Josh daily.

Monday, Josh seemed to be better. He was much more alert. They had taken him off the intravenous feedings, so the bottles were no longer hanging suspended over his bed and he could move his arms freely. Both arms were badly discolored from the numerous injections, the anesthetics, the feedings and the medications he had received; his eye had grown more discolored, too. But he was better able to communicate with us, though still to a very limited degree. He was now sipping liquids by mouth, which was a very encouraging sign that his recuperation was proceeding well.

We asked to see Dr. Crawford. One of the residents told us that unfortunately Dr. Crawford had become ill with the flu, but there were several other neurosurgeons around who were watching Josh's progress. Some of these men we had seen during the period that Josh was undergoing the testing and one or two of them had participated in the surgery. Everything was going well and there was nothing to worry about, we were told, and we accepted these assurances. As it turned out, this was another mistake, another accident of timing that had unfortunate results.

On Tuesday, one of the doctors told us that Josh's progress was such that he might possibly be taken out of Intensive Care the next day and put into a regular hospital room. We were very encouraged—so much so that when we went in to visit with him, I started to explain to him that we were planning to move back to the area permanently. I think he understood me, I don't know; but just at that moment he was gripped, not by a seizure, but by some sort of spasm of all his muscles. His jaw was pulled open by the contraction of his neck muscles, his eyes were forced upward in his head, his entire body became rigid, his back arched. The nurse was right there, and I rushed into the corridor and summoned one of the doctors. They administered some sort of medication. This was what Josh referred to in one of his tapes as the point when he almost lost it all, when he felt that he was truly losing complete control of both his mind and his body. It lasted for several minutes; and I was not able to elicit, from anyone, a specific reason for this. It had evidently been some sort of upset in the brain, probably as a result of surgery.

The next day when we went to see Josh, he had indeed been taken from Intensive Care and put into a regular hospital room. Josh was stronger and better able to speak with us. He said he was hungry but he could not specify what food he wanted. He was not able to identify any food by name, nor could he remember the names of specific items around him. But he could converse with us more normally and was able to respond to simple questions.

We asked, "Are you feeling all right?"

He said, "Yes."

"Do you have any pain, Josh?"

"My arms hurt," he answered. His arms, from the various injections he had gotten, had massive discolorations and a few small blood clots that, I knew from personal experience, would clear up soon.

He was trying to convey some other message to us which took some time to understand. Eventually, he managed to explain. His uncle Ben-Ami had called several acquaintances while he was in Los Angeles and asked them to visit Josh. As a result, a couple of very attractive young women had stopped in for a moment to say hello to Josh and he was very pleased.

The nurse told us that Josh had been helped up on his feet that day to go to the bathroom, which was a good sign, and that his physical recovery was coming along very nicely. Now that Dr. Crawford was ill, however, there was no single doctor attending to Josh. Every now and then one or another of the resident neurosurgeons from the team in charge of Josh's case would stop in for a moment, but none of them seemed willing or able to give us a straightforward answer to any of our questions. They did tell us that the results of the biopsy were not in yet. But all they would say about Josh was that he seemed to be doing all right.

I arranged with a friend to come on Thursday to get our cats and keep them until she could bring them down to Santa Monica to us. The animals were to play an important part in Josh's life after his discharge from the hospital. Our older Siamese cat, Tony, a sealpoint, had been a gift to Josh upon his graduation from junior high school and was an established member of the family. He was very responsive to cuddling and Josh lavished much physical warmth and love on him. Coco, a little chocolate point Siamese kitten, was my Chanukkah gift from Josh the preceding December. She was tiny and very cute, and she was to become a source of particular amusement and pleasure to Josh during the long months of his illness.

On Thursday morning, the movers came. I had arranged to have the cleaning woman there, too, to follow the movers and clean up as they packed and removed items from the various rooms. Her husband came and took some furniture and dishes that I didn't want or had no room for. All the garden furniture and garden tools we just left for the new owners. Everything went very efficiently. They started early and by two or two-thirty they were finished, the truck was loaded and they left. The house was in order. We locked up, saw our real-estate broker, made our farewells to a few other people by phone, and left there for the last time.

We saw Josh late in the afternoon and early evening. Although in some ways he seemed much better, he appeared a little flushed to me and seemed to be uncomfortable. He complained that his head hurt. We waited for one of the doctors to come in for the evening rounds and spoke to him about Josh's complaint. The doctor said he didn't think there was anything wrong. They were aware that Josh had been complaining of headaches, but they considered this normal and were giving him medication for the pain; everything else seemed to be all right. I thought the doctors were being evasive and I was not satisfied with these assurances. Josh did not look as well as he had the day before.

We stayed quite late that evening because Josh was restless and apparently wanted us to remain with him. We spoke with him, told him about the move, tried to keep him amused and entertained. Finally, he fell asleep. They had given him pain medication and a sleeping pill as well. We left about ten o'clock, had something to eat, then went to a motel to spend the night.

Early the next morning we went to the apartment. One of us had to stay there to meet the movers, so Leib went alone to the hospital. When he came back, he said that Josh seemed all right but continued to complain of headaches. Leib had again spoken to one of the residents about the problem and was told that they were watching it and that everything was normal. The headaches he was suffering might be the result of a small blood clot under the scalp in the area of the incision; they would check this out later in the day when they changed his dressings.

Leib went back and forth to the hospital several times during the morning and early afternoon while I stayed at the apartment to supervise the placement of the furniture and the unpacking. I was working at top speed so that the movers would finish as soon as possible and I would be free to go to the hospital to see Josh. As the day progressed and Leib returned periodically to the apartment, he seemed to be more and more upset with the degree of pain Josh was suffering. I, too, became concerned. The moment the movers left, both of us rushed to the hospital.

We arrived just before dinner was served to the patients. Josh was more able to communicate and seemed very pleased to see me, but was suffering considerable discomfort. He complained of a terrible headache. We called the nurse and she in turn summoned one of the doctors. He said he would order a stronger pain medication for Josh, but that everything, as far as he could determine, seemed to be all right. When Josh's meal was brought, I fed him and he was able to eat a little bit.

Aside from the pain in his head, Josh was in a good mood. He told us he had been on his feet that day. The nurse confirmed that they had him out of bed and had walked him down the corridor. We considered this highly encouraging and were very pleased at the progress Josh was making. He had seen himself during the day in the mirror and he asked me about his eye. I realized that he was quite alarmed at the sight of the discolored left eye and the large blood clot which had turned the eyeball red. I explained that this was just the result of the blows from the surgery and that it would soon dissolve. He was much relieved to hear that.

We went home to the apartment that evening. Just a fifteen minute ride! We felt some apprehension about Josh's headaches but were very encouraged by his improved ability to communicate with us and the fact that he had been up on his feet. Although it was still quite difficult for him to express himself, he had certainly made real progress. The exhaustion of the week finally caught up with us and by ten-thirty or eleven both of us were sound asleep.

Starting early Saturday morning, the phone rang almost continuously. Various members of the family were calling for news about Josh. Friends who had found out about Josh from the relatives also called.

After an early breakfast, we went over to the hospital to see Josh. He was in severe pain and was barely able to recognize us. We told the nurse, who answered, "Yes, we know. The doctors are aware of this."

We insisted on seeing a doctor immediately. The nurse left and in a short while one of the residents came in. We told him of our concern, of how uncomfortable Josh was. It was apparent to us that his condition had deteriorated; he only vaguely recognized us and could not follow any sort of conversation. The doctor said that they would check into it in a little while and that we should not be alarmed because logically there wasn't anything, at this point, that could be wrong. Blood clots sometimes formed under the incision and could create a pressure which would cause these symptoms. They had rewrapped the bandages more tightly and this should help dissolve the clot. In the meantime, he had the nurse bring an additional pain reliever.

Being unexperienced in these matters, we had to defer to the doctor's more expert opinion, but we were not reassured. Dr. Stark had said quite explicitly that there would be no pain of any consequence. As the medication began to take effect, Josh fell into a fitful sleep. We gave the nurse at the desk our new address and telephone number and asked her to get in touch with us if there was any change in Josh's condition before we returned in the afternoon.

Back at the apartment, as I started putting things away, Leib and I talked over the situation. We decided that in view of Josh's complaints about the severe pain, it would be better if one of us stayed with him. From what we had seen, the doctors and nurses paid very little attention to a patient's complaints or observations about his own condition; or, if they heard, they seemed not to attach too much importance to them. When we were there, however, greater effort was made to attend to Josh's needs. This is a sad commentary but it was confirmed over many long weeks of observing hospital and medical procedure. Josh's requests or complaints were often completely ignored until one of us was there to see that some response was made.

Leib returned to the hospital and spent the entire afternoon there while I worked at the apartment. He called me at about four o'clock to say that Josh had been dozing on and off fitfully all afternoon but was still suffering excruciating pain, and that he was doing everything he could to get the doctors to come in and take a more serious view of Josh's evident extreme discomfort. I was so alarmed by this, I simply could not stay home any longer but rushed over to the hospital myself.

Josh was asleep and Leib was sitting by his bed. We left the room to talk in the corridor. He had disturbing news. The doctors had been in and had retied the bandage even more tightly around his head while Josh screamed in agony. Although he was not able to carry on any other kind of conversation and appeared to be totally unaware of either Leib's or the doctors' presence, he kept repeating, "It hurts, I can't stand it, it hurts, it's killing me." After rewrapping Josh's bandages, the doctors gave him a large dose of morphine and he fell asleep.

We were very concerned about this development and tried desperately to get more information from the residents. Two of them deliberately avoided us and refused any communication. The one who seemed to have taken charge of the case continued to insist that there was no cause for alarm. "Any severe reaction to surgery, according to the texts, would have occurred within a seventy-two-hour period following surgery. This isn't following that pattern at all. The pain Josh is having now is a full week after surgery so there is obviously no major problem."

This reasoning certainly seemed questionable to us, but then, we were not brain surgeons, we were not knowledgeable about the medical procedures and we had to assume that what we were being told was true.

We went out for a while and walked around Westwood. When we came back at seven-thirty, Josh was still somnolent. We could hear him moaning in his sleep. (Whether he was truly asleep or partially comatose at that time, I do not know; to us he appeared to be asleep.) None of the residents were around, but the nurses assured us that Josh was being monitored very closely; they had orders to administer adequate dosages of pain medication for him to get through the night without any intolerable pain. We really should leave, they insisted.

There seemed to be no way for us to elicit any further information or to get any further attention for Josh, so we went home. We seemed to be on the phone constantly that evening, making some calls but mostly receiving them. Somehow the time passed. Later that night we called the hospital and spoke to the nurse at the desk, who assured us that there had been no change in Josh's condition; he was asleep and there was no need for us to come back to the hospital. Finally, since there seemed nothing else we could possibly do, we retired for the night.

Sunday morning at about eight-thirty or nine, I was awakened by the telephone ringing and I heard Leib talking in the next room. I assumed it was another friend or relative calling to ask about Josh. Suddenly, Leib came rushing into the bedroom, very pale and shaken. "Quickly, quickly, get up," he said. "We must get to the hospital."

A Dr. Burgholz had just called and requested permission to take Josh back into surgery. Leib said, "There's a great deal of swelling in his head and if it isn't operated on to relieve the pressure *immediately*, Joshua is going to die. He's already comatose. I gave my permission." We rushed to the hospital, but by the time time we arrived Josh was no longer in his room. He was down in surgery.

So we had to face another day of waiting. We tried to figure out what had gone wrong. We had been in daily contact with the doctors and nobody had even suggested to us, prior to this emergency telephone call, that we might have to anticipate even the possibility of additional surgery. Leib had only the information relayed by phone and wasn't quite sure of any details. All he knew was that he had given permission for surgery. As he understood it, it had something to do with reopening the area where Josh had previously been operated on and removing the bone flap to relieve the pressure. By the time we got to the hospital there was no one available to give us any further information.

During those hours and hours of waiting in the same awful room, I thought to myself that if in the rush of moving we had neglected to give them our new telephone number, or if for some reason we had gone out early that morning, they would not have been able to reach us. What, then, would they have done? Would Josh be dead now? The doctor had said this was a matter of the greatest emergency, that Josh had to be taken to surgery at that moment or it would be too late. He was that close to death. Perhaps, had they been unable to get in touch with us, it might have been some sort of second chance offered by nature for Josh to be spared an extended terminal illness. Had Leib's response been wrong?

It was a ghoulish speculation, but it haunted me periodically during Josh's next twelve months of agony. I don't think I would have reacted differently from Leib had I been the one to receive the telephone call. I'm certain that the parental instinct forces one to respond, "Yes, go ahead and operate. Help my son, save my son." But again, a crucial decision had had to be made under pressure, with inadequate information, inadequate knowledge of the benefits, dangers, or possible alternatives. At any rate, we had been reached and Leib had given permission for the operation. There was nothing for us to do now but wait.

This operation did not last quite as long as the first one. Josh had been taken down to surgery about nine o'clock that morning, and at four we saw him being wheeled unconscious into the Intensive Care Unit.

We were intercepted by a doctor whom we had seen before but who had not been directly involved with Josh's care during the preceding week. It was Dr. Burgholz, who, apparently, was one of the more eminent members of the neurosurgical staff. Like Dr. Stark, he was a solemn, no-nonsense sort of man. He told us that when he was called that morning by the resident to look at Josh, the edema that had been building in Josh's head had reached the critical point. Josh was comatose. Had the surgery not been performed when it was, Josh would have been dead by now.

The surgery consisted of reopening the previous incision and loosening the bone flap which had been reinserted into Joshua's skull after the first operation. This time the bone section was put in loosely, and it was not secured to create a smooth continuation with the skull. It was raised perhaps an eighth of an inch from its natural seating position and was secured in such a way that if pressure built it could move upward. Then when the pressure went down, it would gradually settle back and ultimately fit almost as well, almost as smoothly as they had hoped after the first operation.

We asked him if this procedure could have been expected, if it was a normal procedure. It seemed to me that he hedged quite a bit on the answer, which was that he had performed such surgery on numerous occasions and that he was considered an expert in the particular technique. A second surgery to relieve pressure was not uncommon; it was done for perhaps one of four craniotomy patients.

I asked, "What happens now if there is any further trouble with the pressure? What can you do then?"

He said, with no more emotion than a discussion of the weather, "There are additional surgeries we could perform. It would require making a new incision somewhere in the skull and removing some portion of his brain. It would be a question then of which function to have removed. It could require creating blindness in Josh, or paralysis, or something else of that nature."

I said instantly, "There will be no further operations. No more! Josh has had enough of this."

It would be intolerable; he would not be a vegetable. He had enough handicaps already. We would not permit any butchery of that type simply to maintain his life further. Since we would not give our consent to any more surgery, it was incumbent upon them now to see that everything was done to restrict further complications, any further building of pressure.

Again, we saw our son in the Intensive Care Unit. But he did not respond to us as he had the first time; he was more dazed. Perhaps he was not completely out of the anesthesia or perhaps he was just more tired. His breathing seemed regular and his pulse was strong. That was about all we could determine. It was terrible to see him back in the same condition of ten days before; it seemed that all the progress he had made had been wiped out.

We stayed very late at the hospital. Not that there was anything more we could do, but we just could not tear ourselves away. We kept popping in and out of Intensive Care just to peek at him, just to see him. Periodically, he'd open his eyes and look at us without recognition. He was flushed and did not appear nearly as comfortable as he had been after the first surgery. We wanted so much for Dr. Stark to be there. Everything seemed to have gone wrong since he had left. Much to our relief, the nurses told us he was due back in the morning. Finally we left the hospital.

We were there very early Monday morning and found out that Dr. Stark had returned the night before and had already issued new instructions. Josh was on a stringently limited liquid intake, literally counted by drops. In addition to the dilantin and phenobarbital that he'd taken since his hospitalization, he was now getting dexamethazone, a cortisone-based medication commonly referred to as Deca-dron. The specific purpose for this new medication was to inhibit swelling and to reduce existent edema.

Josh was more awake than he had been the day before

68

but was still rather flushed and quite uncomfortable. His lips were dry and cracked, and he was asking for water. The nurse told us he was not permitted to have any, so the best we could do for him was to dab his lips with a moistened swab.

Dr. Stark came in to see Josh not long after we arrived. He explained to us about the new medication and told us that Josh would be kept several days with very limited liquid intake to keep down any swelling in the cells of his brain. Although things seemed rather grim and solemn at this moment, with these new procedures there was every reason to anticipate that Josh would recover from this second surgery. He explained to us that even if he had been there, it would have been Dr. Burgholz whom he would have called in for this second operation, since he is expert in the procedure. Although it was unfortunate that there had to be additional surgery, it was not uncommon in such cases. There was now every reason to believe that Josh would be all right—all right in the sense of recovering from the surgery.

We questioned him further about the possibility of additional treatment if Josh should develop more pressure, telling him what Dr. Burgholz said about a third surgery. Dr. Stark confirmed this and said he would absolutely not suggest it—not at this time nor in the future. There was no further sensible choice in surgery; we would just have to depend on other techniques. There was no longer any margin for error.

We described to him, as best we could, the developments during the past week. Although I was sure he had received a report from the medical personnel, I wanted him to be aware of the obviously deteriorating condition that Josh had suffered for so many days before the emergency operation. I felt certain that had he been there, the treatment would have been different. Certainly none of the procedures now being followed had been instituted then. When Josh had first begun to complain about the pain in his head, we saw the residents examine him frequently, but I could not recall one occasion when they checked his eyes to gauge whether internal pressure was building. They simply assumed that the pain was caused by some kind of blood clot under his wound. He was not put on a limited liquid intake, and he did not receive anti-edema medication.

Dr. Stark was in a difficult position. He could not, or would not, say anything more than that the normal procedures had been followed and that it was not uncommon for a second surgery to be required. Still, I felt sure things would have been different had Dr. Stark been there all that time. This accident of timing had cost Josh so dearly. Medical protective ethics stink of patients' blood, pain and death.

For the remainder of Josh's stay in the hospital—a full three weeks more—Dr. Stark never missed a day seeing him. He was even there weekends. Whether this was his normal procedure or not I do not know, but from that time to Joshua's discharge from the hospital, no orders concerning his treatment were ever issued by any doctor other than Dr. Stark.

Within a few days, Josh showed considerable improvement. His liquid intake was gradually increased and, finally, he was again taken from Intensive Care and placed in a regular hospital room. The drama and the horror of the two surgeries were over. His life was no longer in immediate danger. We would enter now into a different phase, a period of recuperation; future treatments would be less dangerous. Now we would retrench. We would begin to comprehend the extent of the damage Josh had suffered and the multiplicity of problems we would be facing with him.

It was two weeks to the day from Joshua's entrance into

the hospital for tests to that dramatic second surgery. Two weeks that completely changed our view of our son, our expectations and our responsibilities. In those two weeks, Joshua went from the wonderfully vibrant and capable person he had been to a severely damaged young man who would have to face the greatest challenge any of us must ultimately confront: accepting one's mortality and preparing to meet death.

Leib spent most of every day at the hospital, more hours than I did because I was busy at the apartment. After Josh was moved back into a regular room and started to feel somewhat better, we began to understand, little by little, what the surgery had done to his brain. He made very slow progress in his ability to convey ideas to us. It wasn't that the amount of information stored in his brain prior to the operation had diminished, but simply that he was unable to summon it at will. The connections in his brain that would enable him to retrieve such information seemed to have been severed.

This was very difficult for us to comprehend. There was no way the doctor could explain it, and over the course of many months, Josh himself, even with the considerable improvement in his ability to communicate that occurred, was never quite able to explain to us what it felt like to know something and yet be unable to control that knowledge or impart it—a computer with some blown fuses. There were also peculiar anomalies in his progress. For example, he had great difficulty in comprehending what was said to him, but his ability to speak returned far more rapidly. Similarly, he was not able to read and could not even recognize letters of the alphabet, but sometimes when he was unable to say what he wanted to say, he could write it. The process was mysterious even to Josh. When he tried to think of a specific word but couldn't say it, if he wrote the message the word would come out quite easily in written form. But once the message was written, he was unable to read it. Sometimes, he couldn't even understand when we read it back to him. He was like a radio system with the receiver broken and the transmitter only partially functional.

During the first week following his second surgery, although there was physical improvement, his mental functioning was blurred. Josh didn't really comprehend much of what was going on, and his ability to understand or appreciate the fact that he had numerous visitors was extremely limited.

In the second week, he started to show real improvement for the first time in all aspects. He was gotten out of bed for short periods during the course of each day to walk in the corridor. His comprehension was improving, although it was easy to see, by his blank expression or his lack of response to certain suggestions we made or questions we asked, that he still had tremendous difficulty understanding us. However, his response to our being there was far more enthusiastic than it had been.

By then he could also communicate well enough to tell us when he was hungry, but he couldn't name what he wanted. After much questioning and guessing we figured out that he wanted some fresh fruit. But he simply could not verbalize the names of the specific fruit. He had a mental image of what he wanted but there seemed virtually no way for him to communicate it.

Gradually, as I gained more insight into the nature of his difficulty, I worked out techniques for helping him. One day I brought him a selection of all the common fruits—banana, orange, pear, apple, tangerine, and so on. I put them before him and he tried to distinguish them by name. We were not successful in getting him to *remember* their names for any period of time, but while they were in front of him and we were discussing them, he could name them and select the one he wanted. The following day I would bring him the fruit he had requested. Usually, he could not remember its name.

One day when I came to the hospital to see him, he gave me a slip of paper on which he had written *macaroni and cheese*. He couldn't read it but he showed it to me and told me that he had written down something that had come to his mind that he wanted to eat. Would I make it for him and bring it to him the next day? I read it back to him and he had absolutely no mental image at all of what it was. The evening before, when he had written the note, he knew what it was he wanted. Thereafter, almost every day, in addition to the fruit, I'd bring him a plastic container of macaroni and cheese. We would also buy him cartons of fruit yogurt, malteds, juices and other items from the dispensing machines.

Like all hospitalized patients who are on the road to recovery, he started asking about going home. He wanted very much to go home. The hospital routine annoyed him; after three weeks there, he was beginning to feel terribly isolated from any normal existence.

Josh was on friendly terms with most of the people who worked on the floor. Some of the younger nurses were cute and he maintained a light, flirtatious tone with them. There were two male attendants who were especially nice to him and he preferred their ministrations to those of the women. He particularly liked to chat for a few minutes each day with the middle-aged man who cleaned the room. Over the weeks this man told Josh all about his family and Josh worked very hard at remembering the names of his children.

But it wasn't all friendly and comfortable. The residents and the interns, in that order, were most intolerable—aloof, pompous, egocentric and generally irritating. There were some nurses, too, who made him uneasy—Oriental girls, particularly the Filipinos, whose accents and unfamiliarity with American idiomatic expressions added to his problems with language. Their attitude was also subtly different. Although they were as attentive as any other nurses, they maintained a certain detachment; they wore the same unvarying expression—a meaningless smile—whether Josh was feeling good or in pain, whether he was getting medication or taking a walk.

On March 7, Dr. Stark said that Josh had been making very nice progress physically and, if all things continued as well as they were going, he would be permitted a short leave from the hospital the next day. Leib would be able to check him out for a couple of hours and bring him home, we could have an early dinner together, and then he was to return to the hospital. It was very exciting for us, and Josh was thrilled at the prospect of being able to leave the hospital.

The next morning, when Dr. Stark saw him, he said that everything looked fine and there was no reason at all why he could not go home that evening for dinner. I rushed back to Santa Monica, went to the market and bought all of Josh's favorite foods and flowers for the table. Josh was always concerned about my physical appearance, particularly since I was indifferent to clothes, so I bought a new pants suit I thought he would like and had my hair cut. Then I went back to the house and started preparing the meal I was planning for Josh's special evening. Leib went to the hospital at three o'clock to get Josh. They were supposed to be home about four. That would give us two and a half hours with Josh.

They didn't arrive at the apartment at four. By four-thirty I was half out of my mind with fear that Leib had had a mishap with the car, or that some other complication had arisen, that in some way Josh had been hurt. It was horrifying the amount of fear I felt, totally out of proportion to the circumstances.

74

Just then Leib called. "We're delayed here at the hospital. Some idiot fouled up Josh's papers for the temporary leave. It's straightened out and we're leaving now. See you soon."

At five o'clock I heard them at the door and I rushed to open it. Josh walked into the apartment under his own power, dressed in slippers, a pair of jeans, his robe, and his stocking bandage on his head. What sheer delight it was to see my son walking into our home—out of the hospital at last.

He came in smiling broadly, but in a terrible state of confusion. Later, Leib told me that on the drive over from the hospital Josh had not been able to comprehend the process of driving or the concept of signs or the idea of direction. What's more, he was painfully aware of this and articulated it to Leib. "I don't know how to explain this, Dad, but I don't understand anything. I don't understand what is happening. I know we are going to the house but I couldn't do any of this."

We were determined to enjoy the fact that Josh was home. We showed him around the apartment and he seemed thoroughly pleased with it. He was delighted to see the cats. He played with them for a while, petted them, and then we sat down for dinner. He ate magnificently, enjoying every bite and in better control of himself and his environment than I had anticipated. The problems he'd been having ever since his surgery seemed much less pronounced here at home. But he did tire very quickly; by the end of the meal I could see he was already wilting and less able to understand us when we spoke to him.

Ever since his first operation, we had tried to do as the doctor had said—to speak slowly, one at a time, and not to jumble conversation. We attempted to keep the conversation on a reasonably adult level, however, and did not speak down to him. I think he appreciated that. He had

75

begun to comprehend, to internalize and to accept the fact that he was having these difficulties in understanding. When he was with us he would not display embarrassment, but rather, when he could not understand what we were saying, would stop us and say simply, "I don't understand," or "Could you repeat that?"

After dinner we sat down in the living room with our coffee. Josh, for the first time, tried to broach new subjects of conversation. He asked his dad about what his plans were. Leib answered that up until this time he had been spending all his time and energy at the hospital and had really not done anything about future plans beyond considering the possibilities. The following week, though, he was planning to speak to various real-estate agencies and then he'd decide where he would work. It was time to start bringing in an income.

We had purchased, in anticipation of Josh's return, a color television set. We turned it on for a while and Josh said he thought it was a very good choice, the picture was clear and the color very realistic. But he was not really able to follow any of the action. When we spoke with him, we were careful to keep the conversation quiet and smooth. We would repeat, with slight variations, whatever message we wished to convey until we could see that he understood. Television, whether it was the news, or a comedy show, or whatever, lacked this repetition; also, there was frequently a confusion of voices. So although he enjoyed the idea of having the color television, he really could not understand it and very shortly asked us to turn it off.

By this time, it was later than we had planned for his return to the hospital. Of course, he had come later than planned as well, but it was time to go. Josh was reluctant to leave, but he accepted the inevitable with good enough grace. We all went downstairs to the car and drove back to the hospital.

76

Josh's recovery was more rapid with each passing day. He was, after all, a strong, healthy young man before this illness and, as damaging as it was to his brain, the rest of his body had great recuperative powers. Even though he had undergone two severely taxing operations, his body was starting to respond very well; his strength was coming back, his appetite improved, his physical coordination was fairly good and getting better. He spent more time now sitting up in bed and walking in the corridors. As a result of his impaired vision he had some difficulty walking without bumping into things, but he was gradually gaining more confidence in his ability to do things for himself. He had a light beard and the nurses had only shaved him once or twice, so he usually looked a bit scruffy. Now he was shaving himself almost daily and looked much better. And the red discoloration in his left eye was fading.

Dr. Stark was anxious to get him started on the cobalt therapy as it was already well past the time he had hoped they would be able to begin. The type of tumor Josh had usually demonstrates an erratic growth, frequently coming in tremendous spurts. Had there not been the complications requiring the second surgery, Josh would have begun cobalt treatments within a week of the initial operation.

The week after Josh had come home for dinner (some two weeks after the second operation) Dr. Stark told us that we would be going down soon to meet the doctor in charge of radiation therapy. We could discuss at that time what the technique involved, what problems we might anticipate, and when the program would be initiated.

In the meantime, Josh was permitted to come home for another evening meal and, again, he thoroughly enjoyed himself. This time he understood far more of the actual trip to the apartment—he wasn't confused by the signs, the traffic or the process of driving. The everyday world in which we function began to make sense to him once more.

Dr. Stark had arranged an afternoon appointment for us to meet Dr. Timmons, the doctor who headed the radiation department. He did not accompany us but told us that Dr. Timmons would keep him informed about Josh's treatment. We went with considerable trepidation but also with the hope that the doctor would be able to give us some encouragement. By this time, a complete biopsy of the tumorous tissue had been accomplished.

Dr. Timmons told us that Josh's tumor was very bad. It was an astrocytoma of two to three degrees of virulence, measured on a scale of one to four (four being the worst). He thought, however, that it was just possible, with any good fortune, that the cobalt treatments could help Josh considerably. We asked if he meant that a cure was possible, which led to a discussion of medical-philosophical semantics. Dr. Stark had been absolutely certain in his prognosis that the tumor Josh had was completely incurable. Dr. Timmons, on the other hand, told us that he looked at it differently. He thought the word "cure" was inappropriate—that if the growth was totally stopped, if the tumor was rendered completely dormant by the treatment, then in his terminology, this would constitute a "cure." In other words, he looked upon cancer as a process rather than a mass of aberrant cells. If the process was halted or interrupted, then, although the portion of the tumor that had not been excised might still remain, if no further changes occurred, that in effect would constitute something in the nature of a cure.

This seemed encouraging to us. We asked him if he had personal knowledge of such a "cure"—that is, a stopping of a tumor of this nature—in this location of the brain. He answered that there were patients he knew of who were still surviving several years beyond what had been anticipated. Although his answer didn't guarantee the existence of a cure, it did seem to give us reasonable cause for hope.

78

Dr. Stark had been so positive in urging us not to think in such terms. And now Dr. Timmons was saying that we could legitimately anticipate not a remission, but a cessation of the growth of the malignancy.

We also discussed at some length what the treatment itself involved and the hazards of cobalt radiation therapy. The treatment consisted of directing cobalt rays through the normal cells of the brain to the area under attack, which in Josh's case was imbedded very deeply, almost in the center of the brain. The radiation to be administered had to be calculated precisely, weighing the possible damage to healthy cells against the amount of radiation that would be effective against the malignancy. There was no way of anticipating exactly what damage would be done, but drawing on many years of case histories and statistical research, Dr. Timmons believed that at this point he could safely administer an adequate dosage to affect the malignancy without significantly damaging the healthy tissues. Josh would go four times a week for up to six weeks, until they had administered to him the maximum total amount they considered safe.

There was, of course, a certain amount of risk. There could be some damage as a result of the radiation, but in view of Josh's condition and the prognosis, this was a risk that had to be taken. A side effect of the cobalt therapy would be the loss of hair from his head, but there was a strong possibility that it would grow back. The radiation might also cause him to feel ill while he was undergoing treatment; one could anticipate nausea and perhaps other side effects as well.

Generally speaking, Dr. Timmons generated an air of enthusiasm and hope, the sense of a real possibility that this cobalt therapy could completely inhibit any further growth of the malignancy. We left feeling very much encouraged. What he had told us gave us reason to be genuinely hopeful for the future.

I say us; actually I mean myself. Leib had never completely believed, up to this point, Dr. Stark's prognosis that there was no possibility of Josh recovering and surviving. Not that he misunderstood what the doctor said, but he could not, and would not, accept all the implications. On one occasion, he suggested to Dr. Stark that the medical profession is subject to error, that there was a slim possibility that the prognosis could be wrong. Dr. Stark agreed that certainly they were not infallible. There are, and there have been, recorded cases of cures or remissions that have no current medical explanation. He did not see this as a possibility in Joshua's case, but he could not entirely rule it out.

I had not shared Leib's feeling. I believed Dr. Stark was totally correct in his prognosis. He was so sure. Also, I had been doing some reading in the literature on the brain and I had not found any cases of cure. Some might live a little longer than others with this type of cancer, but ultimately no one was cured. The tumor's location in Josh's head, the amount that had to be left in the brain, and the degree to which it had infiltrated the healthy tissue seemed to me to indicate a hopeless, irreversible case. Certainly I do not mean to suggest that I reached this conclusion easily, or that it was easy for me to accept, but I felt it was better to be realistic than to live with false hope.

But now, the talk we had had with Dr. Timmons inclined me more to agree with Leib's analysis of the situation—that the doctors do not have all the answers and that just maybe Josh would be lucky and would be one of those who enjoy a near-miraculous cure. Dr. Timmons's positive attitude was so very encouraging, and I so much wanted to believe, that I began to think it possible that Josh might, in fact, recover.

That evening, Dr. Stark told Josh that he would be starting a new treatment to help his condition. He explained that a portion of the tumor had not been removed from his brain, that it was not possible to remove it surgically without creating an unacceptable degree of damage to him, but that it might be safely destroyed by this other treatment, cobalt radiation. We stayed after the doctor left. Because of his difficulty in understanding, Josh had us repeat the explanation several times. I think that by the time we left, Josh had begun to understand the full implications of what we were telling him. The word cancer was never mentioned, nor malignancy, but I could see him absorbing the message.

The next afternoon I took Josh downstairs to have his preliminary examination in radiology. Dr. Timmons was there and another radiologist, Dr. Kalman, who was going to be Josh's personal physician for this portion of the treatment. Dr. Kalman was a young man with fairly long, rather greasy straight black hair and a very dour countenance. He was not at all like Dr. Timmons, who was cheerful and outgoing. The two of them examined Joshua's head, the scar tissue, and checked his eyes for pressure, all the usual things; then they spoke with him about what would be involved. The treatment was not terribly complex; it would require his lying down for short periods of time, as he would to have an X ray taken, and the radiation would be administered by a machine suspended over him. It would take a number of weeks and hopefully it would kill the tumor. Josh accepted this quite well.

Then Dr. Kalman said, "Of course, you know you're going to lose all your hair—but that's nothing very important." With that, the interview was at an end.

I wheeled Josh back upstairs to his room. Josh had been stunned by that last statement. It may seem relatively unimportant to be concerned with the loss of hair when faced with the possible loss of your life. But it was not *just* the loss of his hair. This was the final indignity, the final distortion of his person coming on top of everything else. It had been told to him so abruptly—so unfeelingly. He was sullen and angry.

When we got to his room he said, "Just go away. Leave me alone. You and your operations and cobalt."

When Leib came home I told him what happened. He left immediately for the hospital and I waited at home to hear from him. By eight-thirty or nine I couldn't wait any longer, so I called. Leib answered the phone. Josh was very depressed. He was angry at all the doctors, and he was particularly angry at me, I suppose because I had been the one with him when he was given this awful news. Although he did not, as he had with me, insist that Leib leave, he was uncommunicative and cried to himself. Dr. Stark had stopped by to see him and Leib had told the doctor about the depressed mood Josh was in. The nurses had given him a sleeping pill along with his regular evening medication, and Leib said he'd be coming home soon because Josh had just about fallen asleep.

A few hours later, we received a semi-hysterical telephone call from Simon. Joshua, by some tremendous effort of will, had managed to coordinate all of his thinking powers to enable him, in spite of the fearful difficulty that he had with numbers, to reach Simon in San Diego by telephone. He asked Simon to secure a pistol and bring it up to the hospital so that he could kill himself; he did not wish to live any longer. Simon said that besides calling us, he had already called Dr. Stark but wasn't able to reach him.

Leib and I immediately returned to the hospital. Joshua was wide awake and as soon as we walked into the room, he shouted at me to leave. He did not want to see me. He was so agitated that I thought it best to do as he wished and I left. Leib stayed with Josh to see what he could do to calm him and to comfort him.

I know only secondhand, only from what Leib told me,

what occurred in the course of that night. At this time—
and only this time—Josh gave in completely to despair. He
wept, he shouted, he saw no point in continuing a fight for
life. He made it clear to Leib that he understood how little
he had to look forward to. He was aware that there had
been great damage done to him in the course of the operation and that, even so, the operation wasn't successful. He
knew that his abilities to speak, to read and to comprehend
had been damaged, that he would be disfigured and that
his eyes, too, were failing. Not only was his right eye giving
him trouble, but for the first time he mentioned difficulties
with depth perception and focusing in both eyes. He would
be a retarded freak. And bald! He had reached bottom and
wanted nothing but to die. He had scrawled on a notepad
in bold, black letters, "Kill me, kill me now. I do not want
to live. Kill me now!" He poured out to Leib all his misery,
his frustration, his anger and bitterness and despair.

I don't know just what Leib said to him—he doesn't
remember himself. He sat with our son the entire night,
speaking with him, calming him, listening to him. Maybe
being able to express all that had been building in him for
so many weeks was cathartic for Josh. Maybe Leib was able
to impart to Josh some of his own sense of hope, some of
his own joy that Josh had survived the surgery and had
been improving, and his belief that he would improve
further. Leib refused to accept only the negative aspects
and reaffirmed his determination to believe in the possibility of recovery. In every way possible, he communicated to
Josh his own positive thoughts for the future. And as far as
losing his hair was concerned, he pointed out to Josh that
he had been given incomplete and inaccurate information,
as there was every reason to believe the hair would grow
back. By morning, the worst of Josh's despair had passed.
He had gained a calmness, an acceptance, a new maturity.
Leib saved Josh's life that horrible night.

But Leib came home shaken. It had been a night of intense emotional strain. After he had showered and refreshed himself, we went back to the hospital. Josh was awake. When we came into the room, he didn't ask me to leave. He said good morning. We kissed him and he seemed calm. Dr. Stark came in and checked him over. Josh was a little abrupt with him but courteous. The tremendous emotional blow-up was past.

I believe that if Leib had not spent that night with him Josh might have found some way to kill himself. Such despair must be a rather common occurrence with any patient who has gone through the kind of trauma and disappointment that Josh suffered. In retrospect, it seems to me that it is a problem the doctors should have anticipated. The Neuropsychiatric Institute at UCLA must have people with experience in helping patients to face this kind of depression. Perhaps if Josh had had the opportunity to speak with a psychologist during his initial critical convalescence, this situation might have been averted. I know that his life was in danger that night and that his father saved him. But what if his father had not been there? What if we had not known of the state he was in? None of the medical personnel had reacted in any helpful way.

This was only the first of many problems we were to face as Joshua's illness progressed that should have been anticipated before they occurred. Certainly there are differences in each individual case, but just as surely, there must be some overall pattern to the development of an illness. There must be a reasonable degree of predictability concerning the problems that arise.

We seemed always to be handling problems after the fact, when a little foresight could have greatly eased some of the complications. Moreover, each medical person who treated Josh dealt with a specific, isolated factor rather than with his total being. In this age of specialization, many doctors seem to lose sight of the patient as a person. Maybe the superskills that they develop in limited specialties are ultimately less beneficial to their patients than an ability and an interest in treating a person as the whole, integrated organism he is.

There was never again any reference made to Joshua's crisis of despair. It was not that it was taboo or that we tried to keep him from discussing it. It was just that it was over, it had passed. Josh was again the cooperative, pleasant young man he had been throughout the whole hospital stay.

I accompanied Josh to all of his radiation treatments, both while he was in the hospital and after his discharge. The first one took quite a long time. Careful measurements were made and red lines drawn on Josh's head to mark where the radiation should be focused. They decided to use a technique of alternating the dosage on each side of his head, since the tumor was almost centrally located. The treatment itself lasted only a couple of moments, but the preparations had taken over an hour. The red lines, we were told, were not to be washed off but had to remain there so they could be sure that all the treatments would be precisely focused.

The treatment room was an interior room shielded by thick walls and two sets of heavy lead doors. Josh had to lie on the table with his head at a particular spot, and the machine was swung over his head. All of the control mechanisms were on the outside, and the monitoring was done from outside the room by closed-circuit television. The technicians operating the gear were able to see Josh in the room, and so could I. When Josh came out, he said he had actually felt nothing, that there was nothing to it.

They had given him a very short, small dose the first time. The next day when we went down, they administered the second dose, which was larger. They were to do this two or three more times until they had reached the maximum amount of radiation that could be given at any one time. Joshua seemed to be taking the radiation well, and for the first two weeks there were no side effects. The procedure was not painful, but there was a long waiting period and it was a little depressing having to watch the other cancer patients and their relatives sitting dejectedly waiting for their treatments.

On Friday, March 17, Dr. Stark told us that Josh would be able to go home the next day. I remember the date very clearly because it was to be Leib's forty-fifth birthday. What better present could there have been for Leib than Josh's return?

The knowledge that he was going to leave the hospital really perked Josh up; he was bubbly and excited. He even decided that he was hungry and we took him downstairs to the cafeteria for dinner to celebrate. He wore his robe and his stocking cap, and although people did look at him, he was not such an unusual sight for the hospital. I could see that he was determined to steel himself and learn to live as the recipient of looks of interest or amusement, fear or disgust, rather than the looks he'd lived with all his life until then—looks of admiration or envy, smiling looks, pleasant looks, looks of acceptance.

That evening, when Dr. Stark was by Josh's bed, he took things out of his pockets and asked Josh to name them. This time the little test was not done with written slips of paper; that would have been blatantly impossible for Josh to do. The test was not very successful. I believe Josh correctly identified the doctor's keys and knife, but he could not remember the words *wallet, pen, pad* or numerous other things that the doctor showed him. We didn't make a fuss about it, but it registered in my mind that we would have a lot of work to do to get Josh back to where he could function competently by himself.

Dr. Stark repeated some general instructions about the medications and warnings about getting overtired. Then he asked Josh if he used a water-pik and brushed his teeth very carefully. The dilantin tended to weaken the gums and could cause trouble. Josh looked at him with a wickedly innocent look and guilelessly asked, "Why doctor? Do you mean I'm going to lose my teeth too?" Even Dr. Stark had to laugh.

I didn't sleep all Friday night in anticipation of Josh's return—anticipation mixed with a good deal of apprehension. Only a few days before, Josh had been suicidal. We were now living in an apartment on the third floor. What if another siege of depression should overcome him again? The temptation to jump might conceivably arise and this could be a problem with which I would have to deal. I was also concerned about the medication. In the hospital he was on medication that seemed to be keeping his condition stable, but they also had alternative procedures immediately available in case any problem should arise. Obviously, at home I would not have these alternatives.

It wasn't that I was looking for trouble; I was just trying to anticipate what the possible problems might be so that I could be prepared to cope with them. However, sooner or later he was due home. It seemed to me that it had been forever since he had first gone into the hospital; much more like five months than five weeks. We were very anxious to have him home and although his health was still far from completely restored, if the doctor felt that he was well enough, we would just have to assume that this was so. Of course, the boost to his recuperation from just leaving the hospital, just being back home, should be of great value to Josh. I wondered, watching him over the weeks, whether there wasn't a point in time when a patient could no longer progress in the hospital, just by virtue of its being an institution and so keeping the patient in a mood detrimental to further improvement.

Saturday we went to the hospital in the morning to get Josh. He'd had a last checkup and had been weighed once more just that morning prior to his discharge; he weighed one hundred and sixty pounds, down twenty-five from his normal weight. Although he hadn't requested it, in order to make him feel better about himself, we had brought some of his regular clothing to the hospital and he very happily put on his jeans and shirt. The clothes hung on his emaciated body and he looked even taller than his six foot three inches. Of course he was still wearing the stocking cap and his slippers.

One of the residents came in and spoke to me again about the medication. I had the list of required medicines that had to be given to Josh in six hour increments—every six hours around the clock. This had been stressed the evening before when we had spoken to Dr. Stark. It was absolutely crucial that we maintain this schedule of medication. There might be a fifteen- or twenty-minute time lapse without any undue damage, but as close as possible to a rigid schedule should be maintained. They had also ordered for us a month's supply of medications from the UCLA pharmacy so that we would have a sufficient supply at home to carry us through to the next visit. I carried the large bag of medicines, Leib carried Josh's little suitcase packed with some of his pajamas and toilet articles, and an attendant wheeled Josh downstairs and out the front door to the parking lot. We waited there at the curb until Leib brought the car around. Josh got in the front seat, I got in back and we left for home.

On the way we passed a large record shop which I pointed out to Josh. He asked us if we could stop there for just a few minutes as he would like to buy some new records; he was very anxious to listen to some music again. Of course, at that time, his idea of music was the popular rock bands—things that he had been listening to before his illness. We stopped at the record store and I went in with him. He simply disregarded the stares and walked rapidly down the aisles. He could not read but he could recognize what he wanted by the pictures on the album covers. He picked two or three albums and we left as soon as I paid for them.

During the time we were in the store I noticed that he carried himself very erect, walked confidently and didn't concern himself with the people around him. Like an ostrich burying its head in the sand, he probably felt that if he maintained an unconcerned air others would be unaware of him. A few minutes later we arrived at the apartment. We had brought our son to his new home—his last home.

# Spring 1972

As a drop of water in the sea, as a grain of
  sand on the shore, are man's few days
  in eternity. The good things in life last
  for limited days.
  Apocrypha, Ben Sira 18:10, 41:13

*After they operated on me on the tumor,*
*oh what, what, what, do I want to . . . We didn't know this,*
*they didn't tell me this, my mother and father didn't know.*
*Basically, my memory came back — for a while there, for a*
*couple of weeks — I couldn't talk. I was kind of like . . . I*
*was in Intensive Care, after the cutting they put me in*
*Intensive Care. Well, for a week or two I was like a . . . not*
*a vegetable, my IQ was lovely. It was like in the high*
*eighties, wheeeeeeeee! God it was horrible! I was so sick.*
*Yeah, I was in that Intensive Care and I was really a noth-*
*ingness.*

*I could see, but if I wanted to say anything I couldn't. I*
*tried to say something (it wasn't even a question of saying*
*something simple) it would sound like babooza-za. No mat-*
*ter what I tried to say, it was impossible. I just lay there*
*and each minute seemed like an eternity; oh, it was hor-*
*rible! After quite a few weeks I got out of there and I*
*moved in with mommy and daddy.*

We very quickly settled into a routine
after Josh's return from the hospital. I gave Josh his medicine at two in the afternoon, eight in the evening, and
two in the morning; and at eight in the morning Leib took
care of it. About nine or nine-thirty in the morning I got
up, woke Josh and we had breakfast. After breakfast we
showered and dressed, and on Mondays, Tuesdays, Thurs-
days and Fridays, I took Josh to UCLA for his cobalt therapy. On the mornings when we got off to a fairly early start,

93

we arrived there about eleven. On the days when things went more slowly, or he didn't feel well enough to hurry, we got there at two. No matter what the hour was, there would be a wait. Actually, we had no specific appointment time, so it didn't make much difference.

During the first few months, Josh usually became tired and fell asleep by eleven in the evening. Then I'd have to wake him for his two o'clock medication. But he'd gotten so used to this kind of routine in the hospital that generally he fell asleep again quite quickly. Later, as his pain intensified and he had trouble sleeping, we frequently talked late into the night and he would still be awake at two.

He seemed to have an insatiable appetite, eating huge quantities of food at each meal and snacks in between. He hadn't eaten well while he was in the hospital. But, like most patients who have suffered weight loss during a major illness, as soon as he was out of the hospital and back home he quickly regained his normal weight.

He was feeling better each day, and he wanted to do things, go places. We had to do something to improve his appearance, or at least to make him look less conspicuous. He still insisted on wearing the stocking cap over his head because the area of the scar was fairly tender and he was afraid it might get infected. The best solution we could come up with was to get the kind of large men's knit caps that were popular among the flashier dressers; these were loose enough not to create any pressure on his head and yet still look acceptable when he went out.

At that time Leib had just started working for a real-estate firm in Brentwood. Since he was new and anxious to make some sales, he was always busy on the weekends. Four weekdays were of course taken up with my trips with Josh to the UCLA Medical Center. So Leib and I decided to devote Wednesdays, our only free day together, to taking Josh on excursions. Because Josh's ability to comprehend was still extremely limited, he couldn't do or enjoy anything involving spoken language, such as movies or theater. So we took him to the tourist attractions in the area, which while not taxing his verbal skills, gave him a chance to use the camera he had bought. Although he had a great deal of difficulty in handling the camera, he did manage to take some creditable footage.

The places we visited didn't really challenge him and we maintained an easy and relaxed pace. If he seemed to be tiring we'd stop to eat, or just sit down. Among the places we went were Marineland, the Japanese Deer Park, and Lion Country Safari, which I think he liked best. I can't say that Josh found any of these activities thrilling, but he did seem to enjoy them and they were welcome breaks in the routine we followed on the other days.

About two weeks after the cobalt treatments began, his hair started to fall out. He would wake in the morning to find his pillow covered with hairs; they would fall down his neck, making his back itch and getting all over his clothing. He showered morning and evening but never seemed to be completely comfortable or free of an itchy feeling, and when he washed his hair clumps of it would fall out. He only had a short growth —perhaps half an inch —of hair on his head, because it had been shaved bald for the operation, but even with that, the amount of shedding was formidable. I suggested to him that it might be better to go ahead and shave off what was left, but he didn't want to do that. I think he felt it would keep his hair from growing back. So his bedding had to be changed every day, and he usually changed his clothing and his stocking cap twice a day.

He had been issued about six stocking caps when he left the hospital, and they were beginning to wear badly and lose their elasticity from all the washings. I remember spending one entire day in the hospital trying to get some more. The pharmacy didn't carry them, the in-patient dispensary didn't have them; I couldn't find them anywhere. Finally, I called Dr. Stark's office and explained the problem, and additional caps were then supplied to us. But I was amazed to find that this type of bandage was not available in the hospital pharmacy or any of the hospital dispensaries; nor was I able to find it in any of the local drugstores. Unimportant as they may seem after the fact, little things like this can cause so many problems, so much worry.

Dr. Kalman came to see Josh at the radiation facility at least once a week to find out how the cobalt therapy was coming along. At first, Josh seemed to be suffering no side effects at all, but by the second week, he began to feel a bit nauseous after each treatment. Dr. Kalman assured us that many patients had far more severe nauseous reactions. As the treatments continued, Josh experienced periods of great fatigue, which the doctor assured us was also a standard reaction to this type of radiation therapy and would vanish once the treatments stopped. By the third week, the tiredness grew increasingly worse and he suffered a feeling of general debility, but there was no pain. The only way for Josh to deal with this was to stay at home and get lots of rest.

As the radiation progressed, I noticed that Josh developed a strange odor that was discernible when one was close to him. His bedroom was suffused with it although I kept it well aired and used various room fresheners. It was difficult to describe, although I can still recall it vividly—slightly sour, the smell of something burnt, not an organic material, but rather like the musty odor of a radio or TV repair shop where electronic parts are fused and melted by intense heat. It was apparently a side effect of the cobalt radiation; in fact, Josh may well have been measurably radioactive.

One day when Simon was home visiting he mentioned

the smell to me. He said, "Mom, that's the odor of cancer, isn't it?"

"No, Simon," I replied. "I think it's the cobalt treatment."

"Oh, God—how they're hurting him!" Simon groaned.

The smell gradually declined after the cobalt treatments ended, until finally it wasn't noticeable. But for many months, even up to the day of his death, there was the faintest trace of that odor, just barely perceptible if one was very close to Josh's head.

Apart from the hospital treatments, life was relatively good for Josh the first month or two after his return home. The day he was discharged, we had experienced a strange, new attitude that seemed to overwhelm the three of us, Leib, Josh and myself, on our way home from the hospital. I suppose that it was a tremendous sense of relief that he was finally out, combined with such gratitude that he was alive, that for a short period of time we felt ourselves imbued with a tremendous love for everything and everyone we saw.

Josh seemed to be encircled by a rosy glow. Everything he touched, smelled or saw was a joy, a new gift. He was so pleased with everything, so gentle, so loving, so uncritical, so unwilling to express irritation with anything; it was as though he had not only had the tumor removed but almost as if he had been lobotomized. He was too placid, too undemanding, too indifferent to his own discomfort. This euphoria tapered off, of course. But initially his joy at the gradual return of his ability to walk without bumping into things, to take care of his appearance, to wear regular clothes, to walk outside, to see people, was supreme. He seemed overwhelmed with gratitude to the world simply for existing and for the privilege of participating in that world, to whatever limited degree he could muster.

He tried to express his appreciation in many ways. He

was painfully polite, thanking us for any gesture we made to please him or help him. The first Monday after he left the hospital, he had me stop at a pipe shop on the way home from his treatment and he selected the finest Bulldog pipe the store stocked as a birthday gift for his Dad. The following week sometime, while we were window shopping in Beverly Hills, he bought a bow tie at Saks for Dr. Stark. When Simon came home on one of his visits Josh gave him pocket money. There seemed to be no end to the ways he tried to express his love and gratitude to those of us closest to him.

We had many visitors during this first month or two at home. When his former roommate in Isla Vista came to see him, Josh showed no embarrassment about his appearance or his speaking difficulties. He was a good host but, as with all of the company we had, participated very little in the conversation. We were gradually learning the best procedure to follow when company came. It was wisest to have only a few visitors at a time. Josh would quickly lose the train of thought if more than one person spoke at the same time. He functioned best in a one-to-one situation, so we advised our guests to try to speak to him individually. And when he attempted to carry on a conversation, Leib and I tried to talk as little as possible.

Josh always seemed to enjoy the fact that people were there, but he often found it impossible to follow what was going on. His mind would wander, and he would get a blank look on his face; he would sort of turn himself off. Sometimes, without making anyone feel guilty about it, he would just retire to his room. If someone followed him there and spoke with him alone, it usually worked out much better. If a member of the family or a friend sat with Josh in his room and talked with him for fifteen or twenty minutes, he would really enjoy it.

About two weeks after Josh came home, we celebrated

the Jewish Passover holiday. Josh was well enough for us to take him to the Seder (the special dinner and ritual observance) that his uncle Amnon was giving. It was a small gathering, only Amnon, Marilyn, Leib, myself and Josh, so that he felt quite comfortable. He seemed to enjoy the evening—particularly the fact that it was a formal dinner invitation—and he even sipped some of the ritual wine.

For me, it was an evening filled with symbolism. The thoughts that passed through my mind were really quite natural under the circumstances. If we are indeed God's chosen people, what had God chosen my son for? Moreover, Passover is the story, not only of the exodus of the Jews from bondage in Egypt, but of the sparing of the first-born sons of the Hebrews as well. Did this mean, that my son, coming home at this time, was going to be spared, reprieved from his death sentence? Were we going to be witnesses to a new miracle?

The days were endlessly long. As Josh became physically stronger, his need for activity increased. The Wednesday outings Leib and I took him on helped fulfill this need, but the other six days, except when we had company at the apartment, stretched interminably. I started taking Josh for walks, and sometimes we went to the L.A. County Art Museum or to the zoo. But he still could not watch either television or movies comfortably because of his inability to follow conversations, although this condition improved with time.

During these first four or five weeks at home, I had to teach Josh things that one normally teaches a small child. He had great difficulty with numbers, but he gradually got to the point where, with little hesitation, he could give his address and telephone number to someone and could write his return address on an envelope. The anomaly of his being able to write but not read continued. I had to read aloud to him the mail he received from friends and relatives who could not come to see him. But he was able to answer them himself, particularly if he was relaxed and did not give too much thought to the writing. If he just let it flow, it usually came out with considerable accuracy.

Josh's reading problem became more and more obvious, but when we brought it to the attention of the doctors, they seemed to avoid discussing it. I tried various methods at home to help him. We purchased alphabet flash cards and started working with those, and I also worked out some phonetic word games for him. I got some children's books from the library, but he resented working from them; they were for "kids." I found it was better if I wrote simple stories for him, on more adult subjects, using monosyllabic words as much as possible. His reading didn't improve much, but by the end of April he could read and say the letters of the alphabet about ninety or ninety-five per cent correctly from the flash cards.

I tried to think of some other activity that would not be frustrating for him but that would stimulate his mind. Josh had always been interested in cars and had often mentioned that he was intrigued with the concept of the rotary engine; so I bought him a kit from which he could build a model of the rotary engine. He demonstrated a wonderful determination to function in spite of his handicaps. His hands still trembled, and of course I had to read the directions to him. But he had considerable mechanical skill, so that although he probably understood less than half of what I read to him, he assembled a beautifully functioning model engine over a period of a couple of weeks. He was very meticulous about the construction, and in spite of his trembling hands, there were no spots of glue or misplaced parts.

The model had been a successful venture—it had been very good for the development of his hand and eye coordination and he was pleased that he had been able to put it together. Sometimes, after his treatment, we would have lunch in Westwood and then stop in at a puzzle shop to buy something for him to work with. He had always been extremely good at puzzles, and though he couldn't do them now as fast or as well, he still enjoyed them; they were something he could do that stimulated his thinking but did not involve reading. I also encouraged him to do more filming, and because his hands continued to tremble he bought a tripod to keep the camera steady. I would take him for afternoon drives and if he saw something interesting, we would stop so he could film it.

One especially nice thing that happened to Josh a week or so after he came home from the hospital was meeting Julie. She was a very attractive girl, not much older than Josh, who visited him at the request of Ben-Ami. They had a lovely visit, played records, found that they had many interests in common and she seemed genuinely to like Josh. She treated him as a perfectly normal young man and he responded in kind. There was no expression of pity, which would have been devastating to him; in fact, she was very flirtatious.

I think Josh went out with Julie three or four times during the month of April. She would come and pick him up in her car, and they would go out to a restaurant for dinner or just for a walk and some coffee in Westwood. On one occasion he took her to a movie. He was careful to choose one that he had seen before, and it was a very successful evening. He told me that he wasn't at all embarrassed when she helped him read the menu at a restaurant. She didn't mind and he simply refused to be fazed by the situation. As a matter of fact, he told me, they giggled about it. I was delighted; there could be no better treatment for Josh than to be able to function almost normally with a beautiful young woman.

That same month, about the third week of the cobalt

treatments, Josh had asked Dr. Kalman if it would be all right for him to wear a wig. Josh wanted to be sure that the scar was sufficiently healed so there would be no possibility of infection. Displaying the same want of tact with which he had told Josh that he would lose his hair, Dr. Kalman said, "Oh, yes, I don't think there's any reason why you couldn't get a wig now. Certainly anything would look better than that cap you're wearing."

So we went looking for a wig. I wanted him to get a conservative one, but Josh was adamant. "Look, Mom. I can always tell when someone's wearing a rug and I don't want to look like a geek. I think the only thing to do is to get something really wild and crazy—then I'll look like a college militant, rather than a surgery mutilant!"

Since the neighborhood wig salons carried only conservative men's hair pieces, we decided to look in stores on Hollywood Boulevard; a strange scene for a young man who is not a homosexual, but it seemed the only place where we could find what Josh had in mind. And we did manage to fit him with a frizzy, wild sort of wig that he liked. That evening Josh had a date with Julie. When she saw him in it, she hugged him and told him he looked great, and he glowed with delight.

The wigs (he accumulated several during the year) were a constant problem. Purchasing them was always difficult and embarrassing for us; I couldn't understand why the hospital didn't have arrangements with a particular salon to work with postoperative patients who needed hairpieces. He never felt entirely comfortable in any of them; they ranged from just tolerable to intolerable, depending on weight, the warmth they generated and how much pressure he felt on his flap. As the pressure built and the protrusion on the side of his head rose, the wigs began to cause him considerable discomfort. Finally, in the last months of his life, although his hair had grown back in a strange manner and there were partial, bald areas, he rarely wore one at all. At the moment, however, he was delighted with Julie's response to his appearance and he wore this first rather wild-looking wig when he went out.

After I had taught Josh our phone number and address, we went to re-register to vote because of our move. This would be his first opportunity to exercise his franchise, and he was anxious to establish his eligibility. We found a registrar in front of a large store, an elderly gentleman. Leib and I managed to keep the conversation light and joking so that when Josh was unable to answer the questions properly or made any errors, we could correct them without drawing much attention to his difficulties. Josh managed to sign his name and address correctly and we felt it had gone very well. Later, when our sample ballots arrived in the mail, we applied for an absentee ballot for Josh so that in the primary, with our help, he could fill out his ballot without the embarrassment of being unable to read it in the voting booth.

Josh had his last cobalt treatment on April 20. Generally, he had taken the radiation therapy well. His weight had increased and was practically back to normal, and his comprehension and coordination had both improved noticeably.

Reading, of course, was a severe problem but he had made some encouraging progress. We were feeling very hopeful when we went to see Dr. Stark the following Monday, April 24. Dr. Stark checked him over, examined the scar and flap and tested his reflexes, his vision, the papilledema, and so on. The doctor was pleased to hear that Josh's strength and well-being had improved in so many ways. He decided that we would reduce, in stages, the dosage of Decadron Josh was taking until it was totally eliminated.

This would also reduce Josh's facial puffiness, which had been a side effect of this cortisone-base drug.

We started on the program of Decadron reduction that Monday night. There was an additional reduction on Tuesday and another on Wednesday. Thursday, at nine o'clock in the morning, on the way back to his bed from the bathroom, Josh suffered a severe convulsive seizure. Fortunately, Leib was in the kitchen area adjoining the hallway when this happened. He heard Josh fall and rushed immediately to cradle his head in his lap so that he wouldn't suffer a blow to his head. Leib hollered to me, "Come quickly. Josh is having a convulsion." I was up instantly and rushed out of the bedroom. Without even thinking, I grabbed a wooden spoon from the kitchen to put between Josh's teeth. The seizure lasted quite long. It must have been a full minute before it stopped. Josh was left completely exhausted, somewhere between comatose and asleep. We managed to get him back into his bed and then called Dr. Stark. I reached his secretary, but the doctor was not immediately available. I described to her what had happened and she said she would contact the doctor and would get back to us as quickly as she could.

Josh was sleeping. Leib and I watched him as he lay on his bed. I had never before seen a seizure. The only other convulsion that had occurred at home was the one Leib had seen, the first one Josh had suffered, when he was sixteen. Witnessing it is an unnerving, frightening experience. We tried to keep in mind the doctor's assurances that it is not nearly as bad or dangerous as it appears. This time of course we were more frightened, since any severe blow to the left side of Josh's head could kill him.

Josh was dozing while we sat stricken in the living room. It seemed that all our hope was taken away from us with this seizure. There appeared to be a direct relationship between the seizure and the reduction of the Decadron, as nothing else in Josh's pattern had changed. He had been doing very well until now, but we realized that the internal pressure had not been reduced but was simply controlled by the medicine. Josh wasn't really getting any better.

About an hour or two later, the secretary called back and said she had spoken with the doctor. His advice was just to watch Josh; he didn't think it would require any further immediate attention, but we should see what developed and keep in touch. About three o'clock that afternoon Josh suffered another convulsion in his bed. Something was very wrong.

We called back the doctor's office and were told to bring Josh back to the hospital right away. They were expecting us at the desk and immediately put him to bed in a private room. The young doctor took down the usual, endless case history. We explained carefully, because we felt that it was crucial, the two operations and the recent reduction of the anti-edema medication, and added that there was no longer any margin for further error. We also mentioned how strange it seemed to us that Josh had been put in a room at the end of the corridor, well out of range of the nurse's observation, when it was so apparent that he needed constant monitoring. The doctor thoroughly agreed, and said it was an error but he hadn't known the case history. He immediately arranged for Josh to be moved to a room directly facing the nurse's desk.

They must have given Josh some medication immediately to compensate for the Decadron he had not received during the past two days. He slept quietly. We stayed at the hospital for a couple of hours talking to the doctor and waiting to see how Josh was responding to treatment. At about six-thirty or seven that evening, Dr. Stark came in and checked Josh over. He assured us that Josh would now sleep through the night as a result of the medicines and the extreme exhaustion that follows convulsive seizures.

"What caused the seizure?" we asked him. "Is it some problem resulting from the radiation? Or some postoperative problem? We think it's because the Decadron was reduced."

Dr. Stark agreed. A new buildup of swelling had occurred which he assumed was due to the reduction of the Decadron.

The next morning when we went to see Josh he was sitting up in bed having his breakfast. He felt fine, and had no real recollection of the seizure other than the few seconds of forewarning before the convulsion overcame him. (It is usual, in a seizure, for the patient to have no memory of the convulsion itself.) He did not even remember being brought to the hospital. All he wanted to know now, though, was just how long he would have to stay there. We didn't know ourselves so we couldn't answer the question.

We went back to visit Josh in the early evening, when the doctors usually made their rounds. We were with him when two neurosurgeons whom I remembered well from Josh's previous hospitalization came by. Dr. Stark was not able to be there but they were relaying his findings. Josh would have to continue taking the Decadron. Nothing else seemed to be amiss, and since Josh had been perfectly fine all day, if everything went well during the night, he could come home the next day.

I had stopped at the gift shop on our way in to purchase something to entertain Josh and had found a small puzzle for him. It was just a black plastic box, and the problem was to open it. We brought it upstairs and gave it to him and in about ten seconds he had it open and had put it back together again.

We were joking around with Josh when the doctors came in. After we had talked to them about Josh's condition, I handed the box to one of them and said, "Dr. Garson, why don't you open this?" He looked at it, fiddled unsuccessfully and handed it to his colleague. The colleague also seemed stumped by it and finally put it down on Josh's table. We finished our conversation with them and they left.

Josh and I exchanged looks and he said, "You know, Mom, I haven't been frightened up until now, but if a neurosurgeon can't open that box in one second flat, I may be in very bad trouble." Then he laughed.

He returned home the next day, Saturday, and we had him back on his regular medication. We were to see Dr. Stark the following week to find out what the next step would be. There was no further change in Josh's condition, and everything was now as it had been before—except that we knew that Josh's daily survival depended on his pills.

Our visit to Dr. Stark on Wednesday, May 3, was fairly short as he was primarily interested in seeing if Josh showed any change since his release from the hospital. There was none; the Decadron seemed to have settled that problem. Of course, the implication was there that without suppressant medication a repetition of the edema buildup was possible, and that in itself was a negative sign. At this time, Dr. Stark told us that he had arranged for us to speak with a Dr. Zarinsky, an expert in speech and communication problems at UCLA. We were to see him Friday morning at nine-thirty.

I was very relieved that something was finally going to be done about Josh's terrible problem with reading and comprehension. There had been adequate time, over two months, to become aware of the extent of the problem. I felt, actually, that we should have been doing something about it a lot sooner. My home methods of trying to help Josh had had less than spectacular results and it was important that we attend to this handicap as quickly as possible. None of us can appreciate what a literate society we live in until we lose our reading ability. In order to do the simplest things—such as ordering from a menu in a restaurant, or trying to find out what programs are being shown on television—we must know how to read.

There was one other question that Josh had been anxiously waiting to ask Dr. Stark. Since his first discharge from the hospital, he had been regaining his strength, his confidence, and his ability to function. He now wanted to know when he could start driving.

Dr. Stark was unreceptive to the idea. He said, "Josh, since you had the seizure, I can't permit you to drive until you enjoy one whole year free from seizures."

This was a shattering blow to Josh. I looked at Dr. Stark as he said this, and I sensed strongly that he was telling Josh that he would never drive again.

I understood the doctor's position; it was his responsibility to protect society. If he felt that Josh's driving would pose any danger, however remote, it was incumbent upon him to withhold his permission. But Josh actually posed far less threat than anyone who drinks and drives, or takes drugs or has had a heart attack or is very old. He would certainly have been as safe a risk as half the drivers in this country.

When we left the doctor's office and went home, Josh wanted to discuss this. He felt it was unfair, that it was an imposition of a restriction that would totally handicap him, and he couldn't accept it. It is difficult to explain how important the sense of mobility is to a young person, particularly a California boy who has been driving since he was fifteen. In our society this is equated with manhood, freedom, independence. I made a judgment on my own that I think was not unreasonable under the circumstances, since Josh was so distressed about this restriction. I told him that although I don't normally permit going against the doctor's instructions, I agreed with him in this instance. He must understand, though, that the restriction of his driving was not so much for his own protection, although it was for that, too, but for the protection of others. Surely, he would not want to cause injury to someone else?

"No," he said, "I certainly don't want that to happen."

We compromised. I told him that sometimes, if he wanted to drive, it would be all right if I was sitting beside him. As he improved and felt better, we would then see whether it would be possible for him to drive alone. This wasn't the best solution, but it did partially relieve Josh's anxiety.

Of course, the unspoken part of all this, which was very much in my mind and, I'm sure, in Josh's as well, was that he had never been alone since he had come home from the hospital. Now, after his seizure the preceding week, I would feel even less inclined to leave him on his own. On the other hand, I knew that it was important for him to feel capable of taking care of himself. This was one of the hardest questions we had to deal with. Actually, throughout his illness, I don't think he was ever by himself for more than a few hours. There were several occasions when, to keep him from feeling a prisoner, I deliberately arranged for him to be alone. But I have to admit that during those times I went nearly mad with worry.

Friday morning, we went back to UCLA for our appointment with Dr. Zarinsky—another waiting room, another floor. The doctor was a young man, brusque in his manner and very solemn. Again, we went through the same procedure of relating Josh's case history, an explanation of what had happened and a description of our difficulties. Since his return home, Josh's speech comprehension had improved considerably; the most troubling problem now was his total inability to read. The doctor called in a young woman who was a specialist in testing reading ability and they asked me to leave the room. They spent perhaps forty-five minutes subjecting Josh to various word and letter recognition tests. Then Dr. Zarinsky called me back into the office to deliver his diagnosis. "Your son has a very severe reading disability," he declared, as though he had discovered something that we didn't already know.

We agreed this was a problem that had to be tackled as soon as possible. He told me there was a school affiliated with UCLA and sharing a portion of their campus that specialized in learning and reading handicaps. It was called the Fernald School, and he advised me to call for an appointment as soon as possible. Our best hope, he told us, would be to have Josh start in a program there right away. I thanked him and we left.

As soon as we got home that afternoon I called the school. I explained Josh's condition and mentioned that Dr. Zarinsky had referred me to them. They mailed an application and arranged for me to bring Josh in on Monday, May 15, to begin a program of reading therapy.

About a week after our visit, Dr. Zarinsky called to ask if we'd made arrangements with Fernald. A few weeks later, he called again to ask how Josh was getting along and if we were now receiving financial aid through any agency. This solemn young man, who saw Josh only that one time, was the only doctor during the entire course of Josh's illness who ever initiated a call to enquire about my son's progress or well-being.

The Monday scheduled for his appointment, Josh met his tutor, Barbara Trachtenberg, who was to become very important to him in the months ahead. She worked diligently and kindly with him, yet she insisted that he expend a great amount of effort. The results were not startling, but genuine gains in recapturing his lost abilities were made. In addition, Josh made a new friend and now had a steady activity that gave him some hope and a sense of accomplishment—and brought him into contact with something other than the guarded environment of home, parents, doctor, and illness.

For the first few weeks at the school, he had four hour-long sessions a week. A little later we decided it was better to have him go three times a week with longer sessions of an hour and a half or even two hours, depending on how tired he became; the one-hour sessions had seemed to end too quickly, often at a point when he was starting to make some real progress. Within a few weeks, Josh had mastered the alphabet with assurance and had become reacquainted with the concept of syllables.

*I am having reading problems now. After the operation, besides having physical problems, my memory slips and my head, I've always got a pain in my head. I need to take a lot of aspirin and my whole body is just not working well, shall we say. But at one time I was a fast reader; brrrrrrr like that. My father is just a superfast reader and I caught on from him. . . .*

*We thought that we would give it a little time and things would get better. We hoped that things would get better — we didn't know. I'm talking now about close to a year ago. We didn't know, we got all the bad news later on. At that time, when I got out of the hospital, I . . . we quickly found out that there was some damage there, that I would have to learn to read again. I am very annoyed about the whole thing. As a matter of fact, I think I'm very polite just using the word annoyed, to say the least; I shouldn't use naughty words, but I am pretty angry with Dr. Stark. So it started off and I worked and I worked. Here I was, bright young fellow and I couldn't even read. I worked and worked for days and days and days and days and where did I get? I was trying to say letters like A or P or R. We got a little card book [flash cards] or something,* to read. God, I was having such a heck of a time. I was looking at it and I was just saying to myself, what's this? Or that? Or what's an X? And how do you spell words? One letter words like a or two letter words like go? Couldn't do it! Oh, man, it was not so much frightening . . . but boy was it annoying. Anyway we tried and tried till things got a little better. It was obvious that something more would have to be done. I remember I was still in Intensive Care, I mean excuse me . . . excuse me, I do that all the time . . . "excuse me, excuse me." I'm so polite and at this age, Hah! After I moved into the apartment, we went a couple of times, we went to a bookstore—no a library. . . and practiced to speak [read] words. Gosh, it had been no trouble. I had gone to college and I had been almost a straight A student, like three point eight. Almost all A's. One C. That was the very first semester. You know I couldn't accept that, I always wanted the best. I was going to make it to the top; I was going to be the finest lawyer. We went and practiced on the books, on little kiddie books, on the smallest kiddie ones. It doesn't matter what size they are, but they are little thin books, like, "Run, Spot, run," or "Go, go, go," you know, "I like Jim, I like Sue." There was a little book I'll never forget. It's just in my mind, just a storybook, the name of the little animal was Shadow. It's just kind of a weird thing to think about, but once it got in my mind, because I was having a hard time remembering, when I finally got it, my gosh, it was incredible. I couldn't get rid of it! Shadow.

For several weeks, anyway, I saw that things were wrong, and — so I went to see Dr. Stark, the top neurosurgeon, the one who was supposed to have saved my life. I told him about this other stuff, and he told me, "Why don't you go see a doctor?" Well, anyway, we got ourselves lined up with, and we have been going for many months now, to the Fernald School. It's on the other side of UCLA . . . I go *there to "Fernald University" three times a week for two hours or— What did I say? You see my memory is not so hot . . . I go for a total of six hours in a week and it's, you know, very annoying. But I try to keep my spirits up about not being able to read.*

*Way back when, I could read anything. The books I had to read for college! When I first went up to Santa Barbara, the first quarter, I had four classes. I took a class in, uh— my gosh, it's so annoying when I can't remember the words —I remember, it was atomics. No—Yes, atomics, with the atomic bomb. Yes, I had to take that class. It took a total of ten weeks and in ten weeks I had to read between twenty and twenty-five books for just that one . . . that one class. Can you imagine that? Twenty to twenty-five books, unbelievable! I had three other classes; one was in, uh—uh, what do you call it . . . I'll say one thing—be patient. I'm really getting very tired. Ever since that operation I've got a real worn-out body and my head— OK—history, I took two history classes. Then there was an art class and there was a class in French. Anyway, my gosh, it's annoying when you have problems remembering. I got three A's and a B. I worked really hard, I worked every day of the week. I had to study from three o'clock in the afternoon to about midnight, I really, really worked.*

*Well, anyway, back at Fernald, the school that I go to. At that time my reading was so bad . . . I could see things but to say them was just kind of heartbreaking. Let me say this, things are much, much better. There's, there's a couple of devices to teach people writing [sic] that they have developed over the years. One device is the EDL, another is the Tachette. My teacher is a lovely young woman, her name is Barbara Trachtenberg. She's, it's hard to imagine, she looks like she is twenty-one, maybe twenty-two, but she is really twenty-nine. She really looks young as I am. She is Jewish and just a lovely gal. She is just so nice and patient* and things like that. Anyway, she has been a fabulous help to me. There was this other fellow. He was, his name was Marvin, and he was Jewish also. (I just can't resist the Jewish game there.) He also had very similar problems— surgery, he had a tumor, they had to remove it. He had the same doctor, Dr. Stark. He went to Fernald and he's finally got it together. He's forty, but I swear he looks about thirty . . . I can certainly at this point, I can read anything I want to — It's just a question of time.

With my eyes, I used to be able — I had fantastic eyesight. My eyes used to be more than twice as able to see twice as far away as anybody else. Incredible eyes. I've got beautiful eyes, and they were fantastically strong eyes.

My reading is much better, I can keep it up, but it's hard to read . . . But after the operation, one of my eyes— I can hardly see anything out of it. I can't see the whole thing, I can see a little bit of it. It mixes up with the brain problems that I have so it's hard to see words. I can see short words easily like take, it's easy to see a word like that. Longer words are harder to read. Mentally, I have no problem writing them. When I'm writing a letter I can write and use very long words. No problem with that. But then to go back, to read what I wrote, it's very hard. I have to read it and it takes me quite a long time. I know that may sound a little strange, but no joke, it really is like that.

Anyway, I call the teacher by her first name, Barbara. She's very nice and she's very helpful and she has helped me. Gosh, you wonder, it's been many, many months and you wonder are you ever going to have normal reading back. I'm still a slow reader. When I start out in the morning and, let's say, I've had a good breakfast and I've had a good night's sleep, I'm healthy—had a good lunch and everything, then I go to work at school. Strong, full of strength and all that. After a short time, I start getting tired, physically; it's hard to read. Working on it, it gets *you tired a lot quicker. It would be so nice if I could get that reading back. After the operation there is some part of my brain—they've taken parts out, they've cut them out. I guess by practicing, trying over and over, I'll be able to get better.*

*The mind is the most incredible thing in the world. Unbelievable! There is so much that they don't know; so, so much. They've learned many things but they really have such a long way to go. I mean when they look back a hundred years from now, when they look back, they're going to look at this like, "What's going on here?" So primitive, so archaic. They're almost going to—it's just, I don't want to think of things like that. I mean, it'll be so simple, they'll just touch a button, tell you something and you won't have that pain, you won't have that pain anymore. Save your life? No problem. You won't have a brain tumor —it'll kill it, you just tell it and (snap) it's over, that's what it's all about. It's no joke. I'm not laughing; I'm not crazy. Nobody thinks I'm trying to be funny or anything; they'll have learned an awful lot and things will really start moving. Many thousands and thousands of years ago we animals started out as slow creatures — to high creatures.*

*I guess this whole discussion started — we were talking about this and that, and now we're talking about how it's annoying when I can't remember; talking about how I was able . . . how I was a student. Now I'm a sick nonstudent.*

*I'm trying to get some reading back together again; it's very, very hard. I forget words almost instantly. I'm working very hard but things just flash right away, like you're not going to believe. I'm not saying that I'm not a little bit more tired than I was, than I was an hour ago, true, but it's very hard, it's very annoying . . . You see, I really am having a little bit of a problem, to say the least. Now, I remember!*

*It's very, very frustrating. I have to try and try and things*

115

*that I see right in front of me I always have to say, "What do you call this?" I'm sitting there, I see something right in front of me, I can see it, hold it, touch it, know what it means, but what do you call this? I want to pick up something, to even think of it, to even make something up, it's so hard. And to try to remember it—it's impossible. It's just—that's what I'm trying to say! The fact that you're listening to me and I'm talking is reality. It is unbelievably hard to hold on to memory. It's a little frustrating, a lot frustrating, very frustrating. We think; we use our minds to figure what can be done and we're just kind of—what's the correct word? I mean to say one thing and I wind up saying another, or vice versa. Say one thing and mean another, or whatever, ha! It gets to you!*

*Once in a while I want to say something and it really gets mixed up. I want to start saying something and I realize that I have such bad mix-up in the mind that I have to stop, back up and— listen to myself, to what I said. I'm sure that you people who are listening — will be listening to this recording, understand what I'm trying to say, certainly my mother does. The fact that we've been, it's been almost a year, having to talk to her every day, every day. Can you imagine? From morning to night. We've discussed a lot of these things. I can mean one thing, I can forget it but she understands exactly what I mean. That's really the truth. I'm not kidding you. She knows that, well . . . we kind of joke about it because I mean to say something and I forget what to say or— I say the wrong things. She understands.*

Sometime during this period, we heard about a private cancer clinic in Germany that practiced an unorthodox method involving injections of some sort of tissue cultures made from the patient's own cancerous tissues and also a dietary regime. During the progress of Josh's illness, other treatments came to our attention, mostly through people telling us things they had heard or read. I conscientiously checked each of them out, but we never tried any of these alternate procedures. In most cases the doctors involved stated that their methods had not been tested on brain tumors or had not been successful with them. In the case of the German clinic, my inquiries confirmed that its results were not scientifically well-documented and were of questionable value.

But perhaps the major reason why we did not attempt any of these more unusual treatments for Josh was that he wanted absolutely no part of them. His refusal was based on his awareness of the degree of damage he had suffered. He repeatedly told me that internally, in a way he could not explain, he was damaged beyond repair. He felt that tremendous deterioration was occurring inside his brain and body of which even the doctors weren't aware. If any of the treatments had seemed so promising as to give a real sense of hope, we would have done everything possible to convince Josh to pursue them. Only at the very end did we seriously consider one of these, but by then it was much too late for Josh.

Until the middle of June, we kept to a fairly steady routine. Josh worked terribly hard at Fernald to improve his reading skills and was exhausted at the end of each lesson. The results were encouraging. The process was slow and hard but Josh was very determined. He liked his teacher and they worked very well together. He was really unhappy when the school term ended in the middle of June and he had to wait until the summer session started.

We tried to fill his free time in various ways. Josh had always been interested in his appearance. Now he spent a good deal of time shopping. We never bought much, for it would take him an entire afternoon to find one sportshirt he liked, but it gave us a good excuse for walking on the mall in Santa Monica, looking into various shops, stopping for a cool drink or a cup of coffee. It consumed time, and this was becoming an increasingly difficult problem for us as he felt better physically and had more energy.

It had become apparent to him that his personal friends were going to spend less time with him than he had hoped. This lack of response on their part was one of the most painful aspects of his illness—and he felt much pain. It cut deeper, on a different level, than other hurts he suffered. Although he was always pleasant to them when he did see them and always grateful to receive a letter or a phone call from them, he was sorely disappointed that they came so seldom to visit him.

I tried to think of other physical activities we could do together. We went bowling once or twice, but he was quite uncomfortable afterwards and started to complain of backaches, so we had to give that up. Twice Leib took him out bike riding. They rented bikes at a shop near the beach and rode for a while. Josh seemed to enjoy that very much, but again the back pains proved a problem. Another activity we tried was billiards, which Josh had been pretty good at before his illness. Now with his eye problems, he was not a very good player, and since I had never been good at the game, we were about evenly matched. At first, we played in the recreation room in the basement of our building, but that wasn't very stimulating. Then we started going to a nearby billiard parlor on Wilshire Boulevard, where there were always people around and the jukebox played constantly. Josh liked the lively atmosphere, so we went there frequently.

We also spent a lot of time buying records. At least two or three times a week we would go to one of the large record shops, where Josh would select an album or two. His taste was gradually changing from a preference for hard rock groups to the somewhat softer popular favorites like Jethro Tull, Cat Stevens and John Lennon. He also bought the soundtrack album of his favorite movie, A *Clockwork Orange*, which featured Beethoven's Ninth Symphony. I suggested to Josh that since he enjoyed it so much, perhaps we ought to get some other Beethoven records. Soon he had purchased all the Beethoven symphonies and several sonatas and was now asking me to suggest other classical composers he might like. Soon I began to notice that he rarely played any of his many pop records, but instead would listen endlessly to Beethoven. He also started listening to the FM stations that played classical music. He made a chart of these and the times they came on so he would be sure not to miss the music programs if he was home.

Simon was due home from San Diego in the middle of June. I was looking forward so enthusiastically to his return. He had seen Josh several times since his discharge from the hospital, but he couldn't come very often because he was busy with school, and there was also the expense involved. I wrote to him frequently to keep him up-to-date on Josh's condition and he called often and had long talks with Josh. It seemed obvious to me that Josh was not going to get much better, and in fact there were a number of new developments that I found disheartening. His back ached much of the time and he was having considerable trouble with his vision. The lack of young friends coming to see him was a sad fact in his life, and when his friend Julie went back East, he was left almost totally without young companionship. He was reaching the point where his only association, socially, was with me.

When Simon arrived home, I told him that in my best judgment Josh had only a short time to live, that most likely this would be his last summer. If I was right, it was terribly important that Simon provide for him the friendship Josh so desperately needed. If, as I hoped with all my heart, I was wrong and Josh was going to get better, then he still needed his brother to make the transition. But either way, the logic and demands of the situation indicated that only Simon could perform this tremendously important function of being the best possible friend and companion to his brother for the summer.

I know that Simon intended to do this, that he started out with the most positive thoughts, the best intentions, the determination to be a wonderful buddy to Josh. He told me, "Mom, don't worry about it. I'm going to take over the next few months. Don't you worry. Josh is going to have a great time."

They went out together that first night, and when they came back, not very late, I could see that things had not gone too well. Neither of them was particularly anxious to tell me what had gone wrong, but it was obvious that the evening had been less than successful. I didn't pursue it or press either one of them for an explanation then. They did try again a couple of times—they went to the beach one afternoon, they went to Westwood one evening—but it was obvious to me that there was a problem. Josh no longer responded with enthusiasm to suggestions that they go out together.

Josh told me that the association was not going to be a happy one; that actually Simon's presence at home was disruptive and made him feel uncomfortable. I wanted to explore this further, and Josh finally, reluctantly, told me the primary problem was that Simon seemed to be embarrassed and uncomfortable when they were out together. Simon decided where they should go and when. He was fretful and nervous rather than pleased to be with his brother.

From Simon's point of view, the problem had a different dimension. He tried to accept Josh in his new condition, but I could see he was disturbed by Josh's lack of capability, his difficulty with the language, and his appearance. He couldn't find the right level of communication with Josh and made the mistake of assuming the dominant, big brother role because of Josh's slowness and handicaps.

In July, when Simon announced that he was going back to San Diego to get a job and spend the rest of the summer there, I didn't argue with him at all. It seemed to be the best thing to do under the circumstances. I was terribly disappointed that Simon had not been able to respond to his brother's needs. I had always admired his determination and ability to do anything he really set his mind to, and I felt that in this case his commitment simply hadn't been great enough; he hadn't been generous and understanding enough to overcome the problem posed by the situation; he hadn't put his brother's obvious need ahead of his own distaste and guilt and distress at Josh's illness. Some basic damage occurred to our mother-son relationship with this failure. But the failure was as much mine as Simon's—I expected too much and I had no right to predetermine his ability to cope with the horror that had struck our family.

I know—I knew even then—that Simon tried. He was just eighteen and Josh's illness had been a terrible blow to him. He had identified so strongly with Josh, had so looked up to him and patterned so many of his own interests after his brother's. In school at San Diego, quite unconsciously, he was actually taking most of the courses Josh had taken in his first year at college. Perhaps it was too painful, too difficult for him to see Josh as he now was and still retain a sense of his own future. I don't know. There undoubtedly was some guilt involved. He probably thought he was the only kid who had ever had a death wish about his brother.

*Simon, I think he likes films. He and I always seem to do things like one another. It all started off . . . I'm two and a half years, I'm two and a third years, older than Simon is. He is a little over two years younger and, boy, for brothers, we sure look alike. I mean as close as possible! And we just kind of have a mental telepathy with one another; it's so fantastic, I can't explain it, but he and I know. We've mentioned it to our parents, but he and I know. Many times, so many times, it's ridiculous even try-ing to count the amount of times, we can be driving, whether I'm driving my car and he is on the side, or vice versa, and we're moving, and bam! we snap our fingers, we're going to say the exact same thing at the exact same time. This has happened so many times, it's really, really happened—it's really kind of neat!*

Simon failed his brother, but only because the situation demanded a maturity greater than he possessed. The oppor-tunity passed and never will return. There will be no other chance to spend the summer making his brother's life more bearable. I tried to tell him this. I wanted to spare him the future pain he was creating for himself. My son, my only remaining son, my poor, dear Simon must now live with the fact that he turned away from a situation that he was not big enough or mature enough or unselfish enough to handle. I hope he can forgive himself as quickly and fully as Josh did, and as Leib and I did.

When Simon left, spring was at an end, and summer was upon us.

# The Money Trap

If thou hast not wherewith to pay,
Why should he take away thy bed
from under thee?

Proverbs 22:27

I must interrupt the chronological account of Josh's illness here to discuss the financial aspects of this catastrophe. We may have, because of the peculiarly inopportune timing, been more severely hurt monetarily than other families facing similarly overwhelming medical costs—but I am certain that our case was not unique. It may be a facile statement but it is also unfortunately true that in this country only the very rich or the desperately poor can afford a major illness.

Money, and one's financial situation, probably represent the most sensitive and secretive aspect of our culture. We have recently developed much more open attitudes toward such previously taboo subjects as sex and religious beliefs, but we Americans still guard zealously against any disclosure of our financial circumstances. I am not a stranger to this attitude and it is difficult for me to expose our finances to public view—but it must be done if this book is to help, as I fervently hope it will, in bringing about critically needed changes in our health care practices.

To begin, I should briefly explain our situation when Josh's illness occurred. The preceding summer we had, as a family, made some major decisions and changes concerning our pattern of living. Josh had very successfully completed his first two years of college, and Simon had just graduated from high school and had been accepted at college. For the first time in many years, my husband and I were able to evaluate our personal lives with a view to our own needs and our future. We found that we didn't much like the environment in which we were functioning.

Leib, at forty-four, was working in middle management in the ailing aerospace industry. After ten or twelve years with one company, he had spent the last year and a half bouncing from one position to another, barely hanging on. Thousands of others in the industry were unemployed and seemingly of no further use to our economy; they were too highly skilled, too specialized, too expensive, too old to readapt to industry's changing needs—or so the society seemed to view them. Leib, being less specialized and very adaptable, extremely competent and somewhat underpaid (by relative standards in the industry) was supposedly one of the lucky ones who still brought home a paycheck every Friday evening. But what had he to look forward to? Having stepped back to take a look at our situation, we both recoiled at what we saw.

In searching for alternatives, we decided that we wanted to free ourselves of dependence on industry and to have as much personal control over our economic situation as possible. There aren't too many options open to a man in his middle years, with a family, accustomed to sedentary work and a living pattern predicated on a middle-class income. We decided that real estate would be a fair compromise career and I would work with Leib until he made the readjustment. That decision also helped sever our geographical ties and we resolved, primarily at my insistence, to leave the Los Angeles area, with its smog and traffic congestion, to relocate in one of the most beautiful areas in the world, the lovely small California city of Santa Barbara. To finance this new life of ours, until Leib's earnings could support us, we would have to sell our home and cash in our small stockholdings and insurance. To economize, Josh, who had had his two years away from home at college, would transfer to the University of California at Santa Barbara and temporarily live with us, while Simon would get his chance to be on his own at San Diego State University for his lower division studies.

Having made these decisions, we started immediately to act on them: After a month of study, we secured our real-estate licenses. We went to Santa Barbara one weekend and purchased a pleasant little house. And Leib gave notice at work. So, in August of 1971, we found ourselves comfortably settled in our new home in Santa Barbara. The boys were at home but were set to start school in September, and we had selected a real-estate firm with which we would work. We had the equity in our new house, plus about twenty thousand dollars in cash, and all the confidence in the world that things were going to go well for us.

When that awful February day came, about half our cash reserves had been used up in the intervening seven months; although we had not yet received any return for our tremendous investment in effort, we did have several transactions in escrow which would produce some income. We had reached that point in business activities where we could predict with fair assurance the viability of our gamble.

Simon was apparently doing well during his first semester at San Diego. Josh, at the end of his first quarter at Santa Barbara, had moved into an apartment with some other fellows in Isla Vista. We had helped him a bit financially but by now he had secured student loans and a small scholarship. He had been understandably bored and unhappy living with us, but seemed much happier since his move. In brief, everything seemed to be working out as we had hoped it would. We had less actual security than at any time during the preceding ten or twelve years, but somehow we felt more confident and pleased with our situation.

As with most Americans, particularly the middle-class population, the medical insurance we had carried for most of our married life was group insurance, bought through Leib's company. When he left industry, one of the fringe benefits we no longer had available to us was a group insurance policy for medical coverage. What with the confusion and expense of relocating and the insecurity of our income, we had not substituted any other form of medical coverage. We had it in mind, but were waiting to see if our plans would work out, if we would stay there and continue to function in the real-estate industry.

Shortly before we found out about Josh's illness, perhaps two weeks, we made application for the purchase of family health insurance through a private carrier. Several things became clear almost immediately. First of all, any kind of reasonably comprehensive insurance was very expensive. We had to make some accommodations as a result, primarily in the deductible amount. Still we found that the cost was eight to ten times what the group insurance plan had been, and there was a $1000 deductible amount we would first have to pay before we received any benefits. This, of course, was only for major medical and didn't cover many of the other medical expenses that a family could expect to face.

When we first learned of Joshua's illness, we assumed that since the application for insurance had been made a few weeks before, we would at least be covered for the bulk of the medical expense. During the time Josh was in the hospital undergoing testing, we were contacted by the insurance company and informed that because of Josh's history of one epileptic seizure some five years earlier, he would not be covered by the insurance. The other members of the family would be insured, but Josh was considered uninsurable by current standards in the insurance industry.

For the first time I realized the full implications of any major or chronic illness for a person in our society who wishes to get medical insurance. The insurance companies automatically deny coverage to a person who has a history of any illness of a serious nature. This applies to those who have had, as my son, a recorded incidence of an epileptic seizure, anyone with any history of a heart defect, a person diagnosed as suffering from diabetes, chronic asthma, emphysema, mental illness—the list is endless. Anyone not already insured at the time of the first manifestation of any major or chronic illness will then, for the rest of his life, be uninsurable. In other words, those in our society most in need of medical insurance are not considered safe risks by the profit-making insurance companies and are therefore ineligible for medical insurance.

Ours is the only industrialized country in the world that does not provide some sort of state-controlled insurance for the maintenance of the health of its citizens. The need for some system to make adequate health care available to everyone has become more and more a subject of discussion in our country for the past decade, and there appear to be some strong indications that, in time, some provision will be made for federal subsidization to help meet the ever increasing costs of medical care and attention. It seems to me, however, that there is a stopgap measure that could be instituted almost instantly—one that would create no great confusion and would not interfere with planning for a comprehensive federal system. Just as we have assigned high-risk insurance coverage for accident-prone or notoriously poor drivers, or high-risk fire policies for home protection in brush areas, the government should require every carrier of medical insurance to provide coverage at premium cost for medically high-risk people.

Our financial situation, when we learned that Josh would not be covered by our new insurance, still did not seem bleak. One of the required expenses of his enrollment at the university had been the purchase of a student health policy. So we informed the hospital's accounting department that Joshua was a student at the University of California and carried a student insurance policy. While Josh was hospitalized, we heard nothing further from the hospital about the costs being incurred.

When we checked him out of the hospital, we were

presented with a bill in excess of $10,000, which covered the operating theater, hospital room and medications, but not the anesthetist's fees or the surgeon's bill. The bill was marked "Assigned to Carrier," naming the company that had issued the student policy that Josh held. We continued incurring further costs during the period right after Josh's discharge. Each cobalt treatment was $25; he had weekly blood tests; and we needed more medicines. All of these costs were added to the bill, under the assumption that the insurance would ultimately pay for most of it. The only direct expense we had was an initial deposit of $500 on Josh's entrance into the hospital, and the payments we were making to the doctor.

In May, after these costs as well as the second hospitalization had been added to the initial hospital bill, we were contacted by the accounting department of the hospital to meet with them to discuss the bill. Leib went to the hospital and was told by the person in charge of billing that the insurance carrier had disallowed Josh's insurance policy on the grounds that the illness he was being treated for must have had its origin prior to the time his policy was issued. Well, obviously many illnesses go through extended developmental stages before manifesting themselves. There is no way to know in advance. Certainly we did not anticipate the possibility that Josh had a brain tumor. He had been honest on the application form and indicated his previous treatment for epilepsy, and the carrier had assumed him as a medical risk on that basis. Suddenly, we were faced with the fact that the insurance we thought Josh had was disallowed and we had many thousands of dollars in medical costs for which we were now responsible.

There was no conceivable way for us to pay this amount. Since our return to the Los Angeles area, we had had no income other than what had come to us from our work before the move. From our reserves came the money needed for the move, living expenses, some of the initial payments made to the hospital, the doctor bills we were paying monthly, and the medication we had to purchase out of hospital now that Josh was home. Finally, after several meetings, we arranged with the accounting office to set up a plan of monthly payments, approximately equivalent to car payments, which would extend over the following years. We signed the contract to that effect, and ever since then we have been making these monthly payments to the hospital. We have over ten years left to pay on that bill, and we are still paying surgeon's fees* and making payments on the anesthetist's fees.

There were also the costs of Josh's enrollment in the Fernald School—$9 or $10 an hour for the reading therapy, which he attended five to six hours a week—another bill that was mounting rapidly. Typically, as middle-class people, we knew little about social services available and were thus totally unaware that the financial squeeze in which we found ourselves was primarily the result of either misinformation or a lack of essential information.

The first help we received in handling the financial burden came from Dr. Zarinsky, the reading and speech expert at UCLA. During the interview I had with him, he told me that any extended period of reading therapy for Josh would entail considerable expense. He wondered about our financial condition and what insurance coverage we might have. I told him just what the financial situation was—that Joshua was an uninsured medical patient, that we had incurred enormous bills, and that we were living off our rapidly diminishing savings.

Dr. Zarinsky was shocked that in light of all this we had been offered no help. He assured me there was considerable

* Dr. Stark was most generous in charging what I know must be a fraction of the normal cost for brain surgery of this nature.

assistance available and that we really should have been directed long before this to the social worker (who, incidentally, was hidden in an obscure room, in a difficult-to-find area, on the administrative floor of the hospital).

As people who had always prided ourselves on our ability to provide adequately for our own family, the very thought of anything suggesting welfare or public assistance was anathema. We were exemplars of that great Middle America that in folk myth is self-sufficient, independent, proud. But the fact of the matter was that, as a result of the built-in Catch-22 of the medical insurance setup, we were in deep trouble.

We no longer had any alternatives, and I was reluctantly grateful for Dr. Zarinsky's suggestion that I speak to the social worker. I did so immediately after we had left his office. The only help she seemed able to give us was the suggestion that we contact Vocational Rehabilitation, a state-funded agency. She gave me their address and telephone number, I thanked her, and Josh and I returned home.

It took me about two weeks to make useful contact with them. The woman whose name I had been given was on vacation when I first called. In the meantime, having enrolled Josh at Fernald, I assured them that we would personally pay the costs involved but that we had been recommended to the people at Vocational Rehabilitation. The woman in charge at Fernald agreed with that course of action and told me that they had another student whose training was being funded by Vocational Rehabilitation; she assured me that Fernald would cooperate in every way to facilitate Josh's acceptance.

Sometime in June we were finally contacted to come to the Vocational Rehabilitation offices for an interview. The caseworker there said she felt strongly that Josh would meet the necessary requirements for funding under this program and that as soon as it was possible, they would arrange for the costs at Fernald to be met through Vocational Rehabilitation. She was as shocked as Dr. Zarinsky had been to find that we were attempting to meet all of the costs of Josh's illness with our own very limited financial resources. She pointed out that Josh certainly should be eligible for Medi-cal, a state medical aid program, and referred me to their offices. I filled out all the papers and there seemed to be no question that our financial circumstances, and the fact that Josh was totally dependent on us now for his maintenance, would ultimately qualify him for Medi-cal. This office told me that Josh should also be eligible for Aid to the Totally Disabled (A.T.D.), a county-funded program, which required filling out more papers.

I must say that the caseworkers with whom we had occasion to confer were extremely helpful, understanding of the situation and tolerant of our wish to protect Josh from any sense of being a charity case. It was arranged that Leib and I could fill out the papers and handle all the preliminary red tape. The only requirement that Josh had to submit to, simply to establish his existence, was to be introduced to the caseworker in each facility. We signed releases so that each agency could receive records from the hospital substantiating what we had said about Joshua's illness. We were honest about our financial situation, not making it any worse than it was, but indicating that we were living on diminishing savings and that Leib's current occupation was not yet producing any income.

By the middle of July, we began to hear from the various agencies that Josh had been accepted in each of the funding programs. The problem with these programs, however, was that none provided any help retroactively. If we had not mistakenly believed that Joshua was covered by his school insurance, and if we had filled out a financial statement when he entered the hospital (which the social worker told us should have been suggested by the admissions personnel since we had no regular insurance at the time), the likelihood was that he would have been accepted for funding at an earlier date. If that had happened, most of the medical bills we incurred would have been paid by one or another of the agencies. IF! IF! IF! At any rate, the law did not permit retroactive payment, and Josh would only receive benefits as of July 1, 1972.

From that day on, the schooling at Fernald was funded through Vocational Rehabilitation. The hospitalizations he underwent after July 1, twice for chemotherapy and finally when he died, were paid for by Medi-cal, which in addition paid for two office visits to doctors and two medical prescriptions during any given month. Beginning July 1, Aid to the Totally Disabled sent Josh a monthly check for $118, which was increased to $130 toward the end of the year.

The fact that Josh received this income was very important in maintaining his sense of self-respect. At the time of his first hospitalization, he had a bank account of $700 or $800, which was to have seen him through most of his expenses for that quarter at the university. When he came home from the hospital, he insisted on withdrawing all the money from his bank account and giving it to me. He told me that he would not hear of any other arrangement, that this was to help meet the expense of his illness. Under the circumstances, I felt his desire to contribute to his own maintenance was so important that I finally accepted the money. It was thrown into the hopper with whatever funds we had and was spent along with the rest.

With the checks that Josh received thereafter, which I cashed for him at the bank, he would occasionally purchase gifts for us. He sent his brother some money every time he wrote to him or slipped him some when Simon came to visit. He bought new shirts and pants, most of which he gave to Simon saying they bored him or didn't fit him. He was able, when he went out, to purchase and pay for records he wanted. He would take great pleasure, once in a while, in treating Leib and me to pie and coffee after dinner. If we went out to a movie, sometimes we'd let him buy the tickets. It gave him a tremendous sense of accomplishment to be able to meet his own personal needs and it was a help to us as well.

The Medi-cal was fine as far as it went. With Josh's illness developing, and the increasing side effects, he would average four to five different doctors' visits a month; Medical covered only two visits, but that did mean two less that we had to pay for. As for medication, after the first few months when he started needing additional medicines to treat the back pains, the skin eruptions, the headaches, and other problems, these would average $100 a month, and Medi-cal paid for two of the prescriptions we were constantly in need of. But the primary and crucial help Medi-cal provided was that we didn't have to bear the tremendous burden of the costs incurred by his later hospitalization.

Other treatments toward the end of Josh's illness that were not covered under Medi-cal—acupuncture and hypnotherapy—were a considerable expense. And of course we still had other financial worries and responsibilities aside from those directly related to Josh. But as the year continued and our finances dwindled we became concerned, not about ourselves, but about our ability to maintain a pleasant environment for Josh until his death.

My sister, who is herself chronically ill and in forced retirement living on Social Security, urged us to take her complete savings—$7500 from the sale of her house. We were grateful for this and accepted it with the knowledge that we would repay it in time. My parents, who are elderly and retired, also live on Social Security. The small savings that my father accumulated could, if managed properly, keep them comfortable for the rest of their lives, but he

135

insisted that we use it. I protested that we would only accept his offer as a last resort.

Leib's cousin Judy, herself married to a doctor and thus probably more aware of the problems posed by a major illness, also offered money. So did my friend Charlotte when we gave Josh a trip to Europe for his last, his twenty-first, birthday. With the small amounts that Leib gradually started to bring in, and with the help Josh received from A.T.D. and Vocational Rehabilitation, we managed to continue.

The medical cost bind in which we found ourselves seems, as I look back on it, an unnecessary horror resulting from the absence of an adequate federal health insurance program and, secondly, from errors and oversights by the financial office of the hospital. If there was any doubt at all that Josh's school health insurance might not provide coverage (and the hospital should have been aware of the possibility), we should have been asked to fill out a financial review statement, which would have indicated to them quite clearly, even in the early stages, that we would not be able to handle all the medical costs without receiving some assistance. Dr. Stark must have known shortly after surgery that Josh would need reading therapy, and if we had been helped to arrange that while Josh was still in the hospital, all of the charges would have been handled by Vocational Rehabilitation.

There were other reasons—not only our reluctance, which we overcame, to have Josh apply for assistance, but the fact that such recourse never even occurred to our middle-class minds. We were unaware of any programs of assistance, and no one bothered to tell us of them until we met Dr. Zarinsky. Had he not counseled us when he did to seek the services that were available, I don't know how we would have managed. I don't even know now if there were not, perhaps, other sources of assistance—not only financial, but social or recreational as well—that Josh might have been eligible to receive.

I know that for several months during Josh's early time at home, nothing could have been of greater benefit to him than to be in contact with at least one other person who had gone through a similar experience. I remember asking Dr. Stark during one office visit if he had such a patient who perhaps had made better progress than Josh had done, had regained his abilities to a greater degree, who might be willing to speak with Josh—even if only for half an hour, just so Josh could have some sort of mirror in which to evaluate himself. The doctor's response was quite favorable. He told me that that might be a very helpful idea, that he would give it some thought and see whether it could be arranged. Either he forgot, which I doubt, or he was too busy; perhaps he could not make the arrangements, I don't know, but after his initial response, he never brought it up again and no such contact was ever made.

With the passing of time, I found that I became less willing to ask any of the doctors for anything that might seem to be a form of favor or special assistance, even for routine needs. A resentment was building in me—and an unwillingness that I fought constantly for Josh's sake—to breach their defenses and get behind the fortifications of receptionists, nurses, costumes and customs. Josh's attitudes had also undergone changes as certain aspects of his illness became clearer to him, as his knowledge of impending death became unavoidable. We just let some things drop after having made the initial overtures. How much of this was a result of my own increasing exhaustion with the constant strain of the situation, or a subconscious rejection on my part of what the medical profession has to offer, I do not know.

I cannot fully convey the trauma we experienced throughout Josh's illness: the disastrous results of the tests, the horror of the first operation, the realization that Josh was living under a death sentence, the confusion that followed the second operation, our move back to Los Angeles, the seemingly endless hospitalization, the cobalt treatments. All of these things we coped with and did so, I think, with a reasonable degree of competence.

But if I could have had some other person to give me support in fighting these constant small but important battles, to get access to places, to know of sources of aid, it would have been so helpful. There is a great need in the hospitals for a sort of paramedical ombudsman—someone who, trained to assist the family of a seriously ill patient, is familiar with the problems likely to arise and the opportunities and procedures for obtaining financial assistance, as well as remedial and other services outside the hospitals. I know there are many well-educated women in their middle years who look for challenging and useful work after their children are grown, and I think they might be just the ones to perform this crucial function. With their own experience and knowledge, and perhaps a year of special training, they could serve as mentors and friends to families trying to cope with the catastrophe of a major illness, and guide them in alleviating the patient's fears, problems and complaints.

When Josh died on March 1, 1973, and I wrote the check for the disposal of his body, we had reached the end of our finances. We had not, however, had to compromise on anything that we could possibly give him. What a horror it would have been for him had we not had the resources we did. We were lucky only that while he lived we could provide. For that I am grateful and in no way do I begrudge the drain on our finances caused by his illness. In time, hopefully, we will pay off all the bills. In time, we will regain some measure of financial security. But we learned, through the loss of our son, how little this matters to us.

# Summer 1972

A voice says: Cry out! And I say: What
shall I cry? All flesh is grass, and all its
beauty is like the flower of the field.
The grass withers, the flower fades, when
a wind of the Lord blows upon it.

Isaiah 40:6–8

*The last couple of weeks I've been a little
cocky, a little big-mouth myself. I'm not that happy about
the whole thing, I get a little, you know, a little fresh—
words like that. I see I'm a little loud, I'm a little angry
with my mom and, you know, they try so hard, Mom and
Dad, but they understand, I talk a little too loud. Several
months ago I was a little sweet—a little, I don't know what
the correct term is—I didn't talk loud, I was very polite,
and quiet. Lately I've been just—I've got to raise my voice
just a little bit, just to keep my sanity, cause* WOW, *things
haven't been feeling good in my head—things aren't that
good.*

With the start of summer, Josh was be-
coming increasingly uncomfortable as certain new physical
problems appeared. The backache he had been suffering
from intermittently seemed to become more persistent. In
addition, a rash had appeared on his torso and was getting
worse. We had an appointment with Dr. Stark just around
this time and, after the routine examination, we asked him
about these two new developments. He examined Josh for
both of them but did not say specifically what might be
causing them or, for that matter, what might be done to
remedy the situation. It was obvious that we were now
moving into areas outside his usual area of expertise.

I was beginning to realize that to a man whose skills
were so highly specialized and so much in demand, consideration of these problems was an intrusion on his valu-

able time. It would be better, I thought, if Josh's routine care could be switched to another doctor whose time was less precious and who was more available on a regular basis; Dr. Stark was frequently busy performing surgery or out of town either lecturing or on consultations, and therefore difficult to reach. So I asked him if he could recommend an internist in the immediate vicinity to attend to Josh's peripheral problems. We could give this other doctor a complete history of the surgery Josh had undergone and have him clear any new medications or treatments with Dr. Stark. Dr. Stark was pleased with this suggestion and gave me the name of a local man.

Dr. Grath, whom we saw the following week, seemed to be very cooperative and helpful. I described Josh's medical history and explained that we needed a general physician who would coordinate Josh's medical needs not specifically related to the brain and work in conjunction with Dr. Stark. After the interview, he examined Josh but could not determine what was causing him so much pain in his lower back. He suggested that we have a series of X rays taken at UCLA.

"In a week or ten days," he said, "when I get the results of the X rays and the material concerning Josh's case history from Dr. Stark, I'll be able to prescribe some sort of treatment for the pain."

When we returned ten days later he told us the X rays showed nothing specific—in other words, whatever it was that was causing the trouble was not visible on X ray. However, to help alleviate the pain, he gave us a prescription for APC with codeine which Josh could take as frequently as once every four hours. He also gave us a prescription for Indocin, a tension-reducing drug that hopefully would help eliminate the cause of the backache.

Josh's skin condition just after this changed from what appeared to be a rather minor rash into a full-fledged eruption of acne. His face had literally blossomed overnight into extremely irritating, disfiguring and painful pustules and his torso, both chest and back, was also affected. The doctor said, "This skin problem is not unusual in the case of continued ingestion of cortisone-based drugs such as Decadron. It's an unfortunate, but common, side effect of cortisone medication."

I was a little annoyed. "Why weren't we warned about this possible consequence of the cortisone Josh is taking? Perhaps we could have taken some preventive measures."

"No," he assured us, "there really are no preventive measures. What you should do now is put Josh under the care of a good dermatologist."

Fortunately we knew a fine dermatologist whom Josh had seen on other occasions during his earlier years and who also treated other members of our family. Dr. Marie and Josh had developed a mutual liking, so their relationship was friendlier and a bit more personal than the usual doctor-patient association. The next week Leib took Josh for his first skin treatment. An hour or so after they left I received a telephone call from a distraught Marie, practically in tears.

She told me she had just finished treating Josh's skin condition and that it was rather bad. Although we could not halt it because of the continued use of Decadron, she would do what she could to make it less irritating, less disfiguring. But primarily Marie wanted to tell me how heartbroken she was that Josh had suffered this ghastly illness and surgery. She wanted me to know that he would have her undivided attention at any time he felt the need to see her—either as a patient or just as a friend. She had given instructions to her nurse at the desk that Josh would not require appointments and was to be given priority attention any time he came for an office visit. This proved to be a big help; it was one problem that in the future would be a little easier for us to deal with in response to Josh's needs.

During our next visit to her office, Marie and I had a talk while Josh rested after the treatment. She started by asking me the details of his illness and, after I had explained, she said, "Well, then, the prognosis is guarded."

"No, Marie, not guarded—negative," I replied.

"I've always been so fond of Josh. He had—" she stopped and sighed— "he has such an unusual quality of . . . of promise. You know it's hard to define but there was always more of everything good and attractive about him."

"Yes, such promise. And now—" I lit a cigarette and looked away.

"Look, Marcia, anything I can do, any help I can give— just ask. You know, it's always a sad thing, a shame when this sort of thing happens, but in this case it's worse than that. Josh is such an unusual boy. You know, dealing as I do all day with teenagers and knowing them as I do, it's a double disaster that it had to be Josh, because so many of the others are such absolute shits. Why does it have to happen to the good ones?"

I can't explain how tremendously important it was for me to hear this from another person, one who happened to know my son but was not personally involved. I had had these very thoughts and had been feeling so guilty about them. It was unfair that my son had this heinous disease. I certainly had no other person in mind to exchange situations with him—I wouldn't wish this horror on anybody— but it seemed so grossly unfair, so criminally wrong for my boy to be the one. What a profligacy of nature to have visited this upon a young man with such limitless potential for himself and for society. Why bypass the innumerable young people with none of this potential, the anonymous interchangeables, the replaceables, the ones who would never be able to make any kind of contribution? I thought perhaps there was something basically wrong with me to think in these terms, but to hear the identical feelings stated so positively, so boldly by a trained scientist, a warm and loving doctor who worked with young people because she liked them, was a balm to my burning conscience. I felt so relieved that my feelings had been not inhumane or cruel but on the contrary truly human.

Gradually, Josh's skin improved. It was never again completely clear, but some of the worst blemishes were controlled. Josh was put on a continuing prescription of tetracycline four times daily to reduce the possibility of infection. We also purchased medicated pads, called Tretin A, which helped dry up the eruptions and actually peeled some of the dead skin off his face and body, thereby relieving the disfiguration and discoloration. All these new prescriptions, together with those given by Dr. Grath, almost doubled the volume of Josh's daily pill requirements, which therefore became an even greater burden both in the amounts of medication he had to take and in cost. Josh's back got no better, but at least he was relieved of some of the pain.

As we continued to see the internist, Josh became more and more reluctant about going for the visits. Finally, he told me that he simply could not stand Dr. Grath. I could not imagine why, as it seemed to me that he had been very patient and truly concerned with helping Josh.

"It's not that," my son said. "He gives me the willies. He really scares me."

This was unimaginable to me. After all the horrible treatments he had undergone, during which he had demonstrated no fear of any of the doctors, to have this reaction seemed most peculiar. I asked him to explain further. He told me that the doctor's coldness and his very black and penetrating eyes gave him a sensation of extreme discomfort. I had not been aware of anything unusual about the doctor, but I agreed with Josh in one sense—just as Dr.

Stark was an austere and formal man, this doctor was similarly reserved and formal in his approach. They both epitomized the WASP image—hence foreign to us. However, Josh was so nervous and distressed that I assured him we would try to find some other doctor who would not make him so uncomfortable.

Another doctor was recommended to me by a friend who had recently been seriously ill and had found a very capable internist, who she assured me had a warm and sympathetic personality.

Josh had so many problems; there was so little in his life aside from doctors, pain and discomfort that I thought if a change could be of any slight benefit to him, even a sense of greater comfort, it would be worth the complications involved. To be certain that I was not choosing another doctor Josh might find disagreeable, I arranged for an appointment to speak with the new doctor alone.

My initial visit seemed to be quite promising; Dr. Goldman was talkative and less reserved than the other doctor. We spoke at considerable length about Josh's medical history, about the operation and its aftereffects. Dr. Goldman was apparently knowledgeable about this type of illness. He was positive that Dr. Stark was correct in his prognosis, but he said, "I feel I can be of assistance to Josh in meeting the continuing difficulties he'll be facing. I'll make every effort to create a relationship with Josh that will be comfortable and supportive for the boy."

"That's what we're really looking for. That's what Josh needs," I replied.

I was beginning to feel that we'd found a really human doctor for Josh. Then, at the end of our meeting, I explained to Dr. Goldman that Josh was a Medi-cal patient because of the financial difficulties we had suffered during the course of his hospitalization and our return to Los Angeles. It would be unfair to say that Dr. Goldman blanched, but he certainly became agitated and I could see he was undergoing a considerable struggle. He told me he had had some difficulty collecting from the state on a previous occasion and as a rule preferred not to deal with patients whose medical care was financed in this manner. I gave him my guarantee that should there be any problem with payments from the state, my husband and I would personally undertake to pay whatever charges were incurred. Though visibly concerned about the possible income problems, he consented to take Josh's case.

Perhaps I had hoped for too much. Both of us, the doctor and the parent, were caught up in the Marcus Welby myth that has sprouted in our country, a myth that is continually nurtured and fertilized by the media. Dr. Goldman thought of himself as a doctor whose patients' welfare came first on his list of priorities. Undoubtedly, he envisioned himself as a sorely put-upon, dedicated servant of the sick. Actually, as are most doctors, he was primarily a business-man, and making money is the function of business. I had for a few brief moments hoped we'd finally reached the doctor who would be the wise and wonderful family counselor, ready to offer his strength and understanding to a dying boy. We were both wrong, both bedazzled by the television fairy tales of doctors rushing out to attend, unbidden, their troubled patients. The reality, of course, is that the house call is as archaic as the horse and buggy. Doctors don't initiate calls of concern—these emanate exclusively from patients.

"Ah, well," I said to myself, "so his feet of clay extend up to the navel. Josh will be comfortable with him, and that's all that really matters."

Making this change of doctors was awkward, but when I explained the circumstances to the other internist, he understood and was most gracious. Of course, again records had to be transferred by Dr. Stark's office to the new doctor. As distasteful as all of this was, it was something I had to do to accommodate my son.

By the time Josh went to Dr. Goldman for his first visit, some six weeks or so had elapsed since the original series of back X rays had been taken at UCLA. Dr. Goldman examined him and found nothing visible that could be causing the increasingly severe and frequent backaches, so he ordered another series of X rays. But the results on these were again negative.

Dr. Goldman's best guess then was that the surgery had caused the cancer located in Josh's brain to be seeded or transferred to another part of his body—something that rarely happened. Some of the malignant cells had probably passed down the spinal canal, and he assumed that Josh had now developed a cancerous tumor on the lower spine. Normally, cancer of the brain does not metastasize—that is, travel to other portions of the body—as does, for example, a lymphatic malignancy. But Josh, it seemed, was to be spared no horror. Not only had his brain surgery been unsuccessful, but it probably had resulted in the spread of the cancer. In view of the negative prognosis for Josh's brain tumor, the best we could hope to do in dealing with this new condition was to try to keep the pain controlled through the use of medication.

At about this same time, we received a letter from Dr. Stark stating that as Josh was suffering from a malignant glioma and there appeared to be nothing else that could be done surgically or with cobalt therapy for him, he would like to speak with us concerning another procedure that might prove useful in prolonging Josh's life. What he had in mind was a chemotherapy treatment; although not a curative process, in certain cases it had proven beneficial in retarding the growth of a tumor. He requested that Leib and I contact him should we be interested in discussing it further. He would explain to us personally all that was involved in the treatment and what negative side effects it would produce. Every treatment Josh had previously undergone had created side effects that were, to varying degrees, deleterious. What now?

We arranged for an appointment and early in August Leib and I went to see Dr. Stark. He outlined the new treatment briefly for us. It would involve hospitalization for periods of three days at about six- to eight-week intervals. During the three days, the patient would get injections of an experimental chemical that would as a side effect suppress the formation of white cells and platelets in the blood. Therefore, after treatment the patient would be doubly vulnerable to infection and would have to be more than usually careful of his health. As soon as the blood count returned to normal, in about six to eight weeks, the patient would again enter the hospital for the next treatment. This would be done at least three times. After the third treatment, it could be determined whether it was having any beneficial effect. The chemical BCNU had been experimentally used on animals, and more recently on human beings, for nearly ten years. The statistics indicated that it had some beneficial effect in approximately half the cases and in some of those cases had apparently extended the life span by as much as two or three years. Of course, the results depended on the patient's condition and the actual degree of damage that had already occurred. The treatment itself involved intravenous injections, each taking several hours at a time. There would be nausea, and it could cause some problem with the veins. In addition, since this was still experimental, one of the requirements would be that with each treatment the subject would undergo a series of X rays, brain scans, and an angiogram to evaluate the effect of the chemical.

Dr. Stark told us that Dr. Burgholz, the doctor who had

149

performed the second operation on Josh, was the man in charge of this program, and if we wanted to proceed he would arrange for us to be turned over to Dr. Burgholz. I reminded Dr. Stark how badly Josh had reacted to the angiogram during his original hospitalization, how fearful this procedure had been to him. I told him we would have to think about it before we would even suggest it to Josh. If we did talk to him about it, he would have to be the one to make the decision.

"It is clear, isn't it doctor, that you hold no hope whatsoever for Josh's being cured, or overcoming the malignancy?"

"That is correct, Mrs. Friedman." he replied. "It's just a question of how long we can control the tumor."

"Things get worse with each visit. There's always more pressure and the bone flap is being forced higher and higher," I said.

"Yes. The medications are only partially suppressing the pressure," he replied.

"Well then," I continued, "I have to know what to expect. What is really going to happen to Josh? What must we prepare for?"

"Well that's hard to predict exactly . . ." Dr. Stark trailed off.

"Please, doctor. The truth," I insisted.

Dr. Stark sized us up carefully. I suppose he decided we really wouldn't be satisfied with less than a complete answer. "There are basically three possibilities for the future development of this disease. The first possibility, if Josh is lucky, is that sometime in the future—when, I cannot estimate—Josh will quite suddenly be rendered comatose and will die without regaining consciousness. Another possibility is that the symptoms of brain damage will grow increasingly great. There will be more and more of the same problems with vision, greater difficulty with his speech; his headaches will increase and there could be some paralysis. This could go on for quite a long time. One other possible outcome is that the amount of pressure pushing on the flap will become so great that it will literally tear through the skin. With an exposed wound of that size there would then probably be some externally caused infection of the outer brain membrane which would ultimately lead to complications and death."

I was grateful for the doctor's honesty with us. But what a gruesome litany of possibilities! I asked him, "What if Josh is not lucky enough simply to be overcome with some seizure that will render him comatose and lead to his death? What will you do in the other cases when the pain or the dysfunction becomes too extreme for him to bear?"

He would not answer directly. He said, "We'll do everything we can to relieve his pain. We'll use whatever drugs are necessary—when the time comes."

Needless to say, after that visit with the doctor we were shattered. The only hope—a temporary extension of time —that the doctor had held out to us involved considerable discomfort for Josh and hospitalization, which he dreaded, with small chance of it doing any good. In order to receive even this slim possibility of benefit, he must pay in the one way I knew he would not be willing to pay—by subjecting himself to another angiogram.

Leib and I discussed this for at least a week, whenever we were out of Josh's hearing. We disagreed completely. Leib was all in favor of Josh's submitting to this new treatment. In spite of everything the doctor had said, and in spite of what he saw of his son's development, he still believed there was some possibility of saving the situation. I felt differently. I did not believe there was any chance of Josh gaining an advantage from the treatment. Even if there were to be some small, very short-lived benefit, the outcome would remain the same. I felt it would be an inhuman cruelty to offer Josh the choice of a slim chance of improvement at the cost of so much suffering.

There was another factor that was important in my consideration. As close as Leib was to Josh, and as intimately as we lived with one another—sharing the apartment, spending whatever free time we had together—Josh never felt as free to speak with his father of his feelings about his illness and his future as he had with me. I enjoyed, to a degree I had not been aware of until this awful illness, a comradeship with my son that was unusual. The friendship had always been there and, I suppose, made it possible for Josh to speak with me in a more open manner and about more intimate matters than he would with his father. Because of this, I knew, as Leib did not know or refused to recognize, that Joshua already felt a degree of damage within himself that was not only irreversible and getting progressively worse, *but was unacceptable as it stood.*

Josh had told me quite clearly that if there were to be found a miracle cure that would maintain him in his current state and prevent any further deterioration, he did not consider what he had left an acceptable degree of competence to live a long, useful and productive life. He had first brought this out during a talk we'd been having about the various jobs he'd held before his illness. While reminiscing about them he suddenly stopped, as though a real insight had occurred to him, and he said, "Do you realize, Mash, I couldn't even be a shoe salesman now?"

*Concerning the jobs I've had. The best job I had actually would have been, my gosh, over a year ago, a year and a half ago. Let's see now, it's February, let's say this is February of 1973. It was the summer before. That would have been in 1972. At that particular time, my gosh! time goes, my gosh, I—a year has just been removed.*

I'd forgotten that. Now I know what it was. Last summer was a day like any other day, nothing to really talk about or anything like that because in 1972—why did I get into 1972, that's when I had my operations. Actually it has been a year and half ago since my last job. I had always worked, ever since I was young. I've always kept jobs.

The last job that I worked for was at Bekins. Ha! It was for a man, men who supposedly were just strong bodies and small brains. I don't think I was exactly that case but that was my work. There were two kinds of men. There was one, the big truck-driver, tough guys, and then there were men like me, there were a few of them. I did whatever they told me, and I caught on pretty quickly. I worked there on and off for about six months perhaps, I don't know. It's a system. You learn how to lift certain things in certain directions at certain heights and you do certain things first. One thing I liked about it, it was a rewarding type of feeling because you'd start early, it was fantastic in a way, you'd start early, you had to be there working at seven in the morning, and before you know it the day is over. Just unbelievable, it was so enjoyable.

If I wasn't there on time, oh boy, I would have been in trouble. I would have been fired, just like that! So I made it my business to get up very early. I gave myself an extra hour's amount of time. I'd be all ready—ready to start thumbing a ride at six; I guess I got up around five-thirty or five-forty-five. . . .

I started my work at 7 A.M. and the thing was, it was a job where I really could make money. I've had a lot of jobs over the years, which I'll discuss at least a little bit, but they really didn't pay much money. I don't mind working twice as hard in an hour and making twice as much in that particular hour. Most normal young adults make, in the way of money, maybe as low as the minimum, which would be what? $1.50 or $1.75. At that time, I was making $4.00

an hour at Bekins. Can you imagine that? Four dollars—that is a heck of a lot of money. That's more than I'd ever gotten. Most people, most — Who makes $4.00 an hour? That is you know, top dollar.

When you work at Bekins—you're working physically, but I didn't mind it, I really enjoyed it. There's somebody and—they want all their furniture taken, everything, from the lightest stuff, to the heaviest stuff, and we'd do it. Sometimes, we'd also have to get an extra guy, a third person, but generally two men. It's interesting to a degree. The main thing is that you are busy working.

I myself didn't have any of the responsibility. I didn't have to take any crap, if that's the correct word. All I did is what I was told. Then there's this — the other man. He makes, certainly, a little bit more, but not much more; generally he makes $4.50. He's the guy with the tattoos. All the men who drive those trucks have tattoos and small brain centers. You know, they're not very bright—not super-bright guys.

They have a lot of responsibility besides the work, which he and I both did. He had so much paper work to fill in, you know what I mean, just a — lot of paper work. There's also this little gearing device that checks the time. Anyway it's a lot of work. I'll more happily take fifty cents less than he does and not have any of that work.

The earliest a day can go, the absolute earliest, can be four o'clock. They have a system there and it's this: They have to pay you for eight hours. Instead of you stopping when it's over, the eight hours, they would rather pay you extra overtime. It's overtime and you have to work. That is when your time goes to time-and-a-half. Instead of $4.00 an hour, you make $6.00 an hour. Almost every single time, they'd give me some more work and I'd stay a couple of hours past. We'd normally finish six o'clock. It's a very popular hour, I don't know why, but six is. You'd *really make a good amount of money for one day's work. Now, I think I'm gonna quit, finish with this little discussion, and I'll talk about something else.*

*I once worked—well . . . One day at this other place . . . —I want to say this that while I've been talking, and I've taken the medicine, that pain has REALLY gotten much better. Thank goodness. That pain is so damn ominous, it really gets you. Things are much, much better, I can talk. Anyway, I want to talk about other jobs I've had.*

*Now, before Bekins, the year before I had a job, and— let me remember what it was . . . Oh, yes, the year before that I worked for a clothes store. I worked in the clothes store and — sold people things, and I was damn good at it. I was just very successful. The boss, who was kind of a, I don't want to say anything negative—he usually left. He just went, he and some friends of his, they went out. I don't know the correct word—um, it's the jockeys—the jockeys—you understand why I'm not speaking too good. I'll have to say it this way, this is very archaic but I want to get it out, you know, explain it. There are horses, say ten horses, and there are ten little men, and they race around. OK, whatever that's called—it's a money-making thing, it's for fun. That's where he went often and so there was me and there was an older man who was in charge in the store. We got along very well. We never, in all those months that I worked there, never had an argument. Not once.*

*Now, the year behind—the year behind that . . . I was working, I'd been working for Akron—Akron Department Store. That was a good working store because at Akron it was also one of those jobs where you— It was a combination of things. It wasn't like Bekins, strictly physical work. You had to do SOME work. It wasn't that hard physically at all. You know, you'd carry things — carry things — that's what you might call it . . . Akron Department Store. They* *sell every kind of thing. Regular things, and a lot of Chinese things, yes, a lot of Chinese things. All sorts of Oriental things, Mexican things . . . I think at the time the salary, when I first started that job in 1969, during 1969, I was making $1.00 something—when I left there, it was over $2.00; it was $2.20. Well, anyway, I did a little work there—that was in 1969.*

*I had been working—actually for quite a long time. I'm just talking about those — three important jobs that I worked at. I had some good little discussions over this year when I was with Marcia, thinking about different jobs I had; I had at least twenty jobs since I was sixteen.*

*The first real job I had was at DuPar's—I was just fifteen. I had worked Fridays and Saturdays; definitely every Saturday, sometimes Friday also. Saturdays it was just— what do you call it—where you completely wash something down inside. (My words are not too good; I'm not too happy about that either.) Just the most menial type work, you know, and I don't want to talk too much about that. I was — another word — I can't remember. It's just out of hand, not remembering these words. You understand, you understand what I am talking about. I'm not a nut or anything like that, it's just so hard. That last operation in the head, you know, makes things very hard.*

*Then there was this place called Diamond Jim's, right on the corner of Ventura Boulevard and . . . actually, it's right near where my dad's working now. Isn't that a coincidence? I walked over there because I wanted to get a job. I met this guy there, I thought I sort of knew him, a kid like myself. His name was Claus. As it turned out, we were good friends up until— The last I would have seen him was about a year ago. I haven't seen him in a little over a year. Anyway, we were buddies. Our job was just working in the back room, miscellaneous work, cleaning, whatever you're supposed to do. But they gave us each good steaks. They* hired us and — we worked just twice — I guess we giggled. We had a helluva good time. Anyway that's a job I remember.

I wanted to get a really good, decent job as it was getting close to when I was sixteen. I had my driver's license, I'd be able to drive and everything. So I walked all the way down the Boulevard. I checked every single place, every store. I would go in and say, "Can I get a job here?" I walked miles and miles—finally found a place many, many miles east that was a—place with Italian food. They were closed but I talked to a young fellow there. He was about eighteen and his job was just to sit there and to protect the place. He said that he had a job—in Hollywood. Suggested that I go over to Hollywood and see what's going on. The name of the store was Leed's Shoe Store. He said to go over there and ask them, they might have a job. I went over and met his boss and he said, "OK, when you're sixteen, let me know." It was a week before I turned sixteen.

I started work and it was great. I had just gotten a car. It wasn't a new one, it was my mother's car, a lovely little English car. It wasn't a sports car but it was really cute. It was originally red and they painted it green for me. I drove all the way over to Hollywood. That's about ten miles—maybe a little bit more. It's very enjoyable when you are young and really enjoy driving.

That was in 1967, my first real, mature job you might call it. It was kind of a hard job, in a sense . . . I learned it very quickly. The thing is, when it's shoes, only women's shoes, it's a little hard to learn because there are a million, million shoes there and all they have is just numbers which you must remember. Women sit down and they tell you what they want—a certain kind or style or . . . well, the FIRST thing they tell you is—they don't know what they want! Women are crazy. But they're OK. You have to find their size. Then there's a billion things that they can want

157

*—and when there's two of them! They're talking to each other blah, blah, blah, etc. and they've got tons of shoes, and they go on like that. It's a little difficult to learn, different colors, and there's the whole system. But I did very well; a lot of people just can't learn that.*

*I did well on that job. You can make either a salary or you can raise [commissions] — Anyway, I was making a little over $2.00 an hour. I went to school, but right after school—around noon—I drove over there, and I worked for five hours. Saturday morning, right in the morning, I worked all day till night.*

*A couple of my buddies would get on a bus and meet me there after work. As soon as I would get out, they'd be closing the store, I'd see two of my buddies who had been on the bus — come all the way over there — and then we — we kind of goofed around. At that time, it was extremely exciting. Those guys didn't have cars but I did. Then we'd go back; we all lived in the Valley, right in Encino. I worked there right until Christmastime, 1967.*

*I went to Leed's at Topanga Plaza, which was the complete other side of where we lived, not as far but the opposite side . . . It was much nearer where we lived. It was a much nicer place, I made more money there, everything was better than I could imagine except THAT was the time that I was not feeling well—and I lost my mind and I found out that I had a problem with the mind and all that— I couldn't have any job for a while.*

*So, at that particular moment, I found out— We thought I had—thought that it was epilepsy. Dr. Rubin said "Ah, you've got epilepsy, but it can be controlled." So Gad! It was a shocker. So I didn't have a job for a while as it turned out.*

*In the others [the other tapes] I talked about my tumor; I guess about a week ago I made a recording, which you'll hear. It was not epilepsy as we found out just recently, like a year ago. I never had that, I had a tumor; that's when we had the tumor out.*

*What of little minimal, menial jobs? I had a lot of jobs but they didn't last a heck of a long time. I had a couple that lasted a few weeks—because I was a talker, kept yapping you know.*

*I had one job at a Bullock's department store. My job was—all I was supposed to do was walk around—just walk —in an outfit and see if people wanted anything. There was this little system with little electric lights and if I'd see the light blink and I'd walk over to the phone and I'd lift it up and say, "Yes, yes, what would you like?" One of the chiefs would say, "Go over to . . . This woman wants—" They'd bought something, they're wrapping it up. "She'd like you to take it back, take it over to—take it outdoors and put it in the car." Once in a while, they gave me a tip but you weren't supposed to—and I didn't get many tips. It was a fine job. It was very enjoyable. I liked talking to— There were a lot of chicks—the ones that worked there.*

*There were so many—but they weren't really that important. Let me think if I can think of anything enjoyable, because I had a lot of jobs. I'll talk about a good job at Robinson's department store. That was a fine job. I worked at when I was — in high school — in my last year. School started at eight and I was off at twelve, then I'd grab a bite. I had to be there at one and I worked from one to five.*

*That was a really good job. It was very interesting—very interesting for a guy my age—so young. It was an important job. There was this room, down—in the basement. Inside there they had everything; pens, pencils, any kind of little devices like that, a few hundred different kinds of things. I would only open it for an hour and if people would need something—any supplies—I would ask how* many they would need, and I would give them out, and I would record the numbers and stuff. It was interesting but the place was really a mess. I straightened it out and really did a good job. I had my own desk, special scratch pads and everything. There were just dozens and dozens of different things, and it was a heck of a mess to get that organized. I did that; there were just so many things that I took care of—that I worked on. It was really a top-notch job. Unbelievable, the amount of work that I had to do there, but it was fascinating, doing all those things.

Then it was almost Christmastime and they had an extra —extra amount of things. They needed— Instead of a fellow like me—they needed a full-time man. They said they liked me and they would like to give me something else. The only thing they could get for me at that moment, was, as it turned out, a place where they sold shoes. I knew how to do that and it was fine. Of course I was dressed up. I had to wear a suit, dress very nicely, just like I had before at Leed's in Hollywood. The first few days I did fine—I wasn't that excited with it, but I worked and I got a lot of compliments. Actually, I had to do a lot more paper work, wrapping and stuff, than selling shoes—I started getting bad in my head again so I had to quit that.

But anyway, I thought I'd mention that job. Look at a kid doing that amount of stuff! I really organized things.

I doubt if I'm going to have anything— I'm getting oh so tired. But, wow, I just don't have that damn pain bothering me at the moment. Well, like I said, it must be about two in the morning now . . . I don't have pain—I've gotten rid of that and I am so tired. My reading [speaking] has been— I've been having problems. I explained that before. When you add some extra time to it, it really—really gets you tired out. Anyway, I must have mentioned about eight different jobs I had and, believe me, I had a lot more than that. I know I had at least twenty. It's kind of cuckoo. A couple of times I got fired, but otherwise I would just quit.

Then I did a year of college. The next year I met a really, uh—I was really in love with this chick and I really dug her. I had to get myself a job to be able to stay in San Diego for the summer. Months before school—months before summer had even started—I looked everywhere I could, I tried so hard, everywhere to get a job. Finally, just as school had gotten out, I got myself a job. I had to get a haircut. I had super-long hair, which was unique at that time. Very few had it—and I had real long hair. But I didn't mind—I got that haircut. Also, I had to sell my — sports car, that super-enjoyable Triumph sports car, I really loved it. I had to sell it because, with rent and food—I just couldn't afford everything. It turned out to be a total fiasco —with the girl. I did something dumb. I really liked her but I just made a little mistake. It was so ridiculous . . . Anyway, you gotta learn. So I lost her, and the car, everything. At least I kept the job.

The next year after that—my next job was weekends. I mean I made the money! I worked at Bekins. I quit there because—I had to go up to Santa Barbara. I went up to Santa Barbara and I started my third year of college and that's when the — problems all got started. That's when we found out about the head, and ever since then, well . . . Oh, I think I'm just gonna stop talking now. I'm very tired and it's time to go to bed. So I'll just say good-night mother and good-night father and good-night Simon. Finally going to go to sleep . . . Good-night . . .


I remember trying to encourage Josh when he said he couldn't even be a shoe salesman, telling him recovery would take time, that he was gradually regaining his skills. It was then that he told me how thoroughly ruined he felt, internally. He was damaged beyond saving and he knew it

161

—more clearly than ever the doctors knew. He wanted from us the support we were giving, the concern we were showing for him, the effort to provide whatever help we could for him, but he didn't want fairy tales. He was so grateful that he could speak freely to me, that I was willing to accept openly and honestly the fact that he knew he was dying. He was teaching himself acceptance of death. He was not eager for it to happen but he was without self-pity at the loss of his life. He was working very hard with himself to face the situation honestly, not to play games with himself, and to derive as best he could what benefit life still offered him while facing without regret the fact that it would soon end.

This freedom that Josh felt to speak to me openly about his most sensitive and emotion-laden thoughts had already, on the numerous occasions we spent engaged in long talks with each other, produced several discussions of an extraordinarily painful nature. Josh talked to me about the possibility of his being left, as a result of this illness, in a condition that he would find intolerable. With that inner knowledge he seemed always to have (before the doctors, or we, told him anything of what could possibly happen to him, to his person) he broached to me the subject of a way to handle an unbearable degree of deterioration. He asked me to promise him that if he became paralyzed, or blind, or so unable to communicate that he was in effect helpless, I would do something to end his misery. I assured him that I would—that if such deterioration occurred, regardless of the consequences, I would do something to help him end his life.

I had already been thinking along the same lines. The problem was one of great concern to me because I was so totally ignorant of what one could do and what procedures to follow to assure the desired result with no further pain to Josh. I made my promise to him in good faith; I was totally unconcerned, should the occasion arise, about any punitive action or sanctions that might be leveled against me. But what to do? And how? How useless my education was when any reasonably alert high school kid could undoubtedly specify exactly which drugs, in precisely what quantity, would do the job. And they'd know where to get them, too!

I received a long distance telephone call from an aunt about this time who had within the past two years suffered the loss of her husband. She told me that she had on occasion felt suicidal herself. This opened the floodgates for me and I described the present situation with Josh and the promise I had made to him. I asked her if she could be of any help, and indeed she could. She told me that during one of her periods of depression following her husband's death, she talked to her doctor. As it happened, he was a refugee who had survived a number of years in one of Hitler's concentration camps during the war. He told her that he had secreted upon his person a cyanide pill that could have killed him instantaneously at any time during his long ordeal. In his view, the one factor that had contributed most to his survival during those endless, agonizing years in the concentration camp, had been his knowledge that he had the means to end his situation should the time come when he felt it absolutely intolerable. In his studied view, both as a doctor and as a victim, the important factor in a person's survival capability under extreme circumstances is the knowledge that one still maintains control. In such cases the control consists of the ability at any time to choose self-destruction. As her doctor and her friend, he therefore outlined to her a procedure for committing suicide with an overdose of sleeping pills. He defined the amount that would be needed to do the job surely and painlessly. She, in turn, had found it a great solace to know that she had this alternative, should her depression reach that point.

We had no sleeping pills, but I knew this was a prescription I could easily obtain. I carefully defined to Joshua exactly the procedure to follow if he chose, at any time, to end a situation he found intolerable. If he wanted me to help him in this, I would. If he wanted to do it himself, whenever he chose to, that was perfectly acceptable. We would not love him any less nor lose any of our tremendous respect and admiration for his courage and his dignity. I assured him that in my view it was both acceptable and correct that he should have at his command the opportunity to decide that his pain or unhappiness was beyond his strength to bear. I promised him as soon as it could appropriately be done, I would get him a prescription for sleeping pills.

I had never before seen such an expression, both physical and verbal, of gratitude on the part of my son. It was as though a tremendous burden that had been torturing him had been removed. This willingness on my part to understand his need and accommodate it had returned to him the one thing he had to have in order to tolerate the loss of everything else he suffered—power over his own life. Josh never chose to employ it. I never thought he would. But his security in the knowledge that it was available to him was undoubtedly the greatest gift I was able to give him during that last year of his life.

Josh also spoke to me during this period about the disposal of his body after death. He asked me if it would be all right to arrange for his body to be cremated. He considered this a dignified and appropriate procedure and said that it would relieve us of the feeling that we were tied to any specific piece of ground or that we had a responsibility to come periodically to visit a grave. He was not a bit maudlin or overly solemn about all this, merely concerned in a practical way that I make these arrangements for him. I promised him that everything would be as he wished.

All these conversations with Josh were factors that entered into our discussions concerning the new treatment, chemotherapy. Finally, Leib and I reached a compromise decision. I would write to the doctor, and if we could elicit from him a promise that the angiogram would not be a requirement of the treatment—in fact, that it would not even be mentioned—then we would broach the subject to Josh. I can't recall the letter in all its specifics, but I know I reminded Dr. Stark that the first angiogram had hardly been productive—that it had indicated Josh's tumor was encapsulated, on which premise he performed the first operation, a false premise, it turned out, since the tumor proved to be widely infiltrated throughout Josh's brain. Its accuracy as a diagnostic technique thus left a good deal to be desired. I also recall stating that I understood these testing procedures were a concomitant part of the chemotherapy treatment and contributed to the accumulation of statistical data, the *sine qua non* of scientific research. Although normally this might be good science, in a case such as Josh's, however, where there had been such an intense reaction to the angiogram, surely it could by no stretch of the imagination be interpreted as good medicine. Therefore, I asked him if he could get a guarantee from Dr. Burgholz that this procedure would be completely omitted from both discussion and actual testing. In time, I received a letter concurring with our request. We then arranged an appointment for the end of summer to bring Josh in to speak with Dr. Stark concerning chemotherapy.

The summer was not all doctors and medicines and pain. Actually, with the use of codeine when necessary, Josh was able to enjoy various activities at this time. Three days a week we went to the Fernald School for his lessons. Although the lessons were just two hours long, somehow they busied the whole day. The mornings were taken up with washing up, getting dressed and breakfasting. While I made the beds and did the dishes, Josh usually devoted some time to playing with our cats, particularly Coco. He had taught her to retrieve paper balls and she would return them to him no matter how many times he threw them. Frequently, she'd initiate the game by bringing him scraps of paper she'd tear from the newspaper. The lessons at Fernald were in the early afternoon. By the time Josh finished he would be a little hungry, so we'd have a late lunch in Westwood and then do some window shopping or perhaps visit a relative.

Usually on the other two days, sometimes on the weekends, I would take him to the beach. He loved the sun. The tan he developed, in addition to the treatments he was getting from Dr. Marie, considerably improved the condition and appearance of his skin. As the summer progressed he looked much better. His weight had stabilized at about one hundred and eighty-five pounds, the same as before his surgery. His hair had started to grow back in a most peculiar manner; there was a wide strip of growth perhaps four inches wide, from the center of his forehead to the back of his neck, but the sides of his head were bald. Gradually, over many months, more hair grew forward over his temples and across the back of his head, but there remained a bald patch on each side approximately three inches square where he'd received the most direct exposure to the cobalt. Josh didn't want to wear his wig in the sand, so he would leave it in the car when we walked on the beach. We'd try to find a relatively isolated spot and as soon as I spread the blanket he'd lie down and close his eyes. He never watched the young people fooling around in the water or on the sand. He didn't observe the boys'showing off on their surfboards. His wet suit hung unused in his closet. The normal beach activities of his contemporaries were no longer available to him, so he closed his eyes and his heart to these painful reminders of his deprivation and merely absorbed the sunshine.

During the summer Josh's cousin David, who had been working out of the city, came back to town and on several occasions came to the apartment and took Josh out. One Sunday afternoon they went to a museum; another Sunday, they went to a young people's concert in Santa Monica. A couple of times they went out to movies in the evening. These activities were a big boost to Josh's morale, but unfortunately, David did not stay long in Los Angeles. When he left to take another job out of town, that area of social contact was again cut off for Josh. I believe once during the summer his cousin Fabe's wife, Sheila, came over and took Josh out for the afternoon, but Fabe did not come. I tried several times to suggest that Fabe and Sheila invite Josh to their house when they had some young people over, but they chose not to. I did not pursue the idea beyond a certain point—not with Josh's dignity and self-respect as a constant example to me.

Josh did try to make contact with some of his old acquaintances in the area. He called another friend named Larry, whom he had known from childhood. They had not been intimate friends but they had known each other for so long and had kept in casual contact over the years. Josh asked him to come over and they went out to lunch. After that he never saw Larry again. The only further contact they had was when Josh called to ask him over for another visit, but he never came.

Josh also tried to contact his friend Lee. He found out from his mother that Lee was in Seattle, so he wrote to him there. It was a painful letter and difficult for him to write. He tried to keep the tone light but yet to communicate clearly what had happened to him. The response Josh got was a letter that was a garbled mixture of obscenities concerning rip-offs, brutal sexual encounters, and an offer to go into business together. Lee wanted Josh to supply drugs from Los Angeles so he could peddle them in the Seattle area, where they were in short supply and would bring in good prices. It was a shattering experience for Josh to receive such a venal response to his overture for friendship and communication without one reference to his illness or his condition.

These two unrewarding efforts to re-establish links with old friends, coupled with the obvious absence of his two best friends, must have discouraged him from making any further gestures toward the young people he knew in Los Angeles, as he never tried to reach any others. But he did maintain close contact during the summer with some of his older relatives. He made it his business to speak with each of them at least once weekly by telephone, and whenever possible we would have them to our place or visit their homes. These became, for the rest of his life, his only physical social contacts. He maintained a correspondence with his two best friends. Once or twice his pal Larry called him long distance and that was a real treat for Josh. Julie, too, had kept in touch by mail and phone. Josh told me that she was having emotional problems and looked to him for help. He offered what advice and counsel he could, but as the months passed and his condition worsened, he told me apologetically that he didn't have the strength left really to assist her. Strength to help her? I never could understand from what hidden reservoirs he kept summoning the courage to suffer his own anguished existence!

*I do like my relatives. There is—when it comes to the elderly people that are relatives, blood relatives, that's the correct word—there's Henry and Bessie. I*

168

*love them. There's Adina, she's uh the other one [grand-parent], uh, the other—her husband died a couple of years ago.*

*I like the elderly people. I talk to elderly people. I seem to have learned so much since I came out of that hospital, almost a year ago. I didn't feel like a twenty-year-old, a twenty-one-year-old, and I don't feel like a forty-year-old, I just feel like a learned person. I feel like I'm higher up in the sky, you know, I see things with perspective . . . I don't know, my age feels different. I love talking to older people.*

*I don't particularly like teenagers. I don't like children or people that— Young ages are very—they can be selfish, very cruel and hard, you know. As people get older they get, not only smarter, wiser, kinder with age, but they be-come learned. It's not the other way around. People don't start off at a certain age and start working backwards as they get older, start learning less; certainly not. As they get older they learn more, and more, and more. I love talking to older people. They've learned more, and they talk more, and I listen to what they have to say.*

*The young crowd, twenty-year-olds, they become cocky; very often have big mouths and it's not enjoyable. I'll say it again, I do like talking to older people.*

*Now let's see, in relatives, well I'll certainly have to talk about that. I don't know but — I get — you know — I get things mixed up. Cousins—I always get that mixed up. It's so hard. My cousin's uncle's son's cousin! That's been something that's been such a real bother for me. It's so hard to keep it organized.*

*Anyway, there's Anna, she's Henry's sister, yeah. She's seventy-two, she'll be seventy-three sometime during the year. I mean, she was born in 19—1900. So was my grand-mother, so it's easy to keep up with her. It's real good, 1900. Anyway, there is Anna and her son. There are two boys; one of them that's unimportant, the other one's name is*

Babe. It is very interesting. I was told this before I had my tumor operation—she has a brain trouble. They found this out at least a year and half or two years ago. I didn't know that I'd be winding up with a tumor myself. Before— See, things get a little mixed up . . . I didn't even know her that well. She was a cousin or whatever the term is [great-aunt] but she was a nice woman. So she feels— It varies—she loses her memory — so do I. There was one point where I was at my worst—my real worst—and then I started to get better — and she started getting worse; things were about equal. Anyway, now, she gets worse and better, worse and better, but she's never ill—like in very bad condition. She's not feeling that good though, and now she has a nurse. Her whole mind is a little mixed up, she really doesn't function, it's horribly sad. I feel pretty bad, that she's in so bad a shape. I talked to her all the time. I used to see her once a week. At the moment, I see her once every two weeks or so, two and a half weeks, three, I don't know. I see her a little bit less. I'm not so happy myself; I'm not feeling too good myself. . . .

Talking to her doesn't really help me one bit; I help her, or I try. We don't . . . talk about these things because she's really not in a talkable condition — I understand things; my problem now is trying to explain things, using the correct words, and stuff like that. But my mind is OK. I don't know if I lost anything, or how much, but I had the brains then and I've got them now; maybe a little cut up, a few pieces out . . .

I'm changing my discussion to mention some other things.

We live in Santa Monica—we go to Westwood. I used to go very often, I used to like seeing it. Now, I'm getting kind of bored, I've seen it so many, many times. We live almost at the beach. We live on Euclid, Euclid is the street, and we live twelve streets from the water — on the beach, the California side of the world—

*I'm really tired, man, I've got to get some sleep, I'm almost worn out. But I really love my mother and my father and Simon; he's really a good kid. Good-night . . . Good-night.*

Brain research indicates that the two hemispheres appear to serve largely different functions. When one hemisphere is damaged, however, the other has the capacity to compensate for the damage and to take over certain of these functions. The left hemisphere, where Josh's damage occurred, houses the centers of communication, language, comprehension, reading, speech, and so forth. The right hemisphere supports more nonverbal, aesthetic capabilities. This seemed to be very clearly demonstrated in Josh's case. With the decline in his communicating abilities, his other more sensitive and artistic interests became far more dominant. I have already mentioned that he became suffused with a gentleness and loving feeling toward all life and was far less stubborn or argumentative than he had previously been. He could not tolerate violence, whether on the screen or witnessed personally. Many of the news broadcasts on television became so painful to him that he would leave the room.

His interest in classical music grew tremendously. He had become quite familiar with much of Beethoven's music, and as we purchased more records he soon began to enjoy Brahms, Schubert, Schumann, Mozart, Mendelssohn, Bach and Mahler. His tastes seemed to lean heavily toward the German composers. We tried some Russians, but the only one he liked was Tchaikovsky. He liked Dvořak, particularly the *New World* Symphony; Sibelius turned him off, but Grieg was fine. We kept experimenting and he was very excited and eager about expanding his knowledge and enjoyment of music.

One Sunday Amnon, Marilyn and Josh's grandmother took him to the beach for a picnic. In one of the small shops along the beachfront he found a plaster bust of Beethoven which he bought for his room. I knew from the many trips we'd made to art galleries how much he admired the work of Salvador Dali, so I ordered a lithograph of El Cid for him; it came during the summer and I hung it in his room. My sister Ruth gave him a simple sketch of a head by Picasso. The whole tone of his interests was changing, becoming far more sophisticated aesthetically.

A couple of times during the summer I took him to concerts in the Hollywood Bowl. These were nice evenings for him, but as the summer progressed and the pain in his back became more severe, he found the walk from the parking lot to the stadium more difficult and the uncomfortable seats too tiring. By the middle of August we reluctantly decided to forego any further outings at the Bowl.

Before his illness, Josh had been such an active, lusty, physical young man. Although now the quality of his activities was different, and his pace was extraordinarily reduced, like a wound-down record, he still wanted to do something almost every evening. Frequently we went to the movies. His comprehension had much improved but it was still far from normal. As an example, his reactions to two science-fiction films we saw differed tremendously. With just one or two whispered explanations from me, he was able to understand *Silent Running* with no trouble at all and he enjoyed it immensely. But *The Andromeda Strain* was completely beyond his ability to follow and was thus a frustrating rather than an enjoyable experience. This alerted me more than ever to the fact that I had to be very careful in what we selected to see, so as not to remind him of his reduced capabilities.

Though I often suggested that Leib and he go out together alone, Josh would insist that I accompany them. Once in a while, however, they would go by themselves and these were the rare times that I would have a few hours alone in the evening. Joshua's pace was such that I was constantly fighting to adjust myself and my normal patterns of movement to his greatly reduced speed. It was as though Josh functioned in slow motion. Everything he did took an inordinate amount of time. His morning shower and shave and dressing could take up to an hour and a half. He was at this point in his illness still capable of doing almost everything, but at slower speeds. This was extremely difficult for me, and I was perpetually exhausted throughout Josh's illness.

The constant emotional stress, combined with the physical restraint, left me enervated. Any activity that was not directly related to meeting Josh's needs became impossible for me to do. It was very important to me to be in contact with my friends, with other people that I knew, with normally functioning society. I did not want to be isolated, to be reduced to a total and exclusive involvement with Josh, but it was physically impossible for me to summon the additional energy needed to initiate even a phone call to someone else. I was always pleased when someone called me, but if I had a moment free, a moment that was not devoted to Josh, I would use it to try to consolidate what energies I had left.

A terminal illness creates in both the patient and his family great emotional needs for contact with people involved in normal activities, with interests other than medical. When Josh first entered the hospital, and shortly after his return home, we constantly had company. But as time passed and the need for social contact actually increased, the degree of contact diminished—not so drastically for me as for Josh. I have heard from many other people that this seems to be a pattern in such situations. I wish it could be changed, that people could be made aware that though the immediate postoperative time may be dramatic, the patient's need for company is far greater when the excitement and confusion have passed and the brief future stretches into bleak routine.

On the evenings when we didn't go to a movie, Josh and I would often go to Westwood, walk a little bit and stop in one of the cafes there to have either coffee or a cool drink. It was so unutterably sad, our being there surrounded by young people: boys with their girlfriends, groups of young men, clusters of girls—and poor Josh with his mother. I know how much it pained him to observe the young people around us living a life no longer within his reach. Gradually, I think he came to accept the fact that he was truly comfortable only with me, because I fully understood his needs and his limitations. He was above all else a realist, so he made do with what was available.

Once or twice a week, we would go out in the evening to the local family pool parlor, a bright and lively place. Josh would pick out some songs on the jukebox, we'd have a beer, and we'd shoot a few games of pool. Gradually, it became more difficult for him to bend over the table, and although we continued this activity throughout the warm summer months, I could see as time went on that it became less enjoyable for him.

During August, Josh purchased a lovely little American Indian turquoise and silver pendant which he gave me for my birthday. At the same time, his grandfather gave him a watch with a band that had turquoise insets, and I bought him a turquoise ring. It wasn't the specific objects involved, it was the exchange of love, of concern and interest. Josh derived such joy from giving and receiving gifts.

We had not seen Simon since he had left in July, and Josh was becoming quite concerned about him. He usually telephoned fairly regularly to speak to his brother. Josh told me, "You know, Mom, Simon's basically a good kid. I'm not angry that he couldn't stay here."

I remember one evening as we walked in Westwood, Josh had been talking about Simon and all the experiences he had yet before him, his future, and what he would do. He paused and with the sweetest smile he said, "You know, Mom, if this tumor had to happen to someone, I'm so glad it was me and not Simon. He couldn't have handled it."

Toward the end of August we decided, at the insistence of my sister and my parents in Sun City, that as a change for Josh, we would take him there and leave him overnight for a visit. Leib and I would go on to San Diego to see Simon, and the next day, on the way back, we would pick up Josh and return home.

We found Simon in good shape. His busboy job in a large motel was physically very taxing but paid enough for him to support himself. He was sharing a house with two other young people, he looked reasonably well, and his room was clean and orderly. We had a fairly good visit although there was, on my part, a certain constraint. I was pleased of course that he was demonstrating a maturity and ability to handle his own life and manage without any financial assistance from us, but I still felt that his real place was at home with his brother. I wonder now, in retrospect, how much of that feeling was selfishness on my part. Did I just want my burden eased? Josh had been so much more understanding of Simon and willing to accept his love at a distance, if that was what his brother could give.

When we picked up Josh the next day, he told us he had had a fine visit. Ruth had done everything possible to entertain him. They'd gone to a small local fair and then out to dinner, and at her insistence Josh had done all the chauffeuring. She gave him a necklace that she had made for him and a finger weaving for his room. It was a good change but it had all been a strain. He was glad to be getting home.

. During the summer, particularly on the evenings when Josh and I went places close to home, I would let him drive. He was, as he had always been, an extremely competent driver. If there was any change now, it was that he was doubly cautious because of his awareness of his impaired vision. A few times that summer, I could see his sense of frustration building at having to depend on me to take him places and do things with him. One day he challenged me, in the sense of confronting me with his determination for independence. He announced, "I'm taking my own car and going out somewhere—by myself."

I think I rather surprised him by readily acquiescing, but I felt it was the only appropriate response. It was obvious to me that he was constantly exercising restraint, muffling his irritation and anger at his helplessness and the constraints of his condition. His self-control, his lack of self-pity were demonstrated daily to a most remarkable degree. He had to rebel a little bit; certainly this was a small demand for him to make. I often thought if it was me, I'd just say to hell with it all and do something crazy. But Josh had too much love and concern for us to do that. By his example of controlled acceptance he was teaching us how to tolerate his death.

I doubt whether, on this or any other of his solitary drives, he ever went more than the five or six blocks to the mall in Santa Monica. There he would park and go for a little walk before returning. Usually he'd bring back a small gift for his dad or for me. Each time he went for a drive, and it was only a few times, I would wait on the porch of our apartment, imagining with terror the infinite number of problems that might arise. As soon as I saw his car coming down the block, I would go back into the apartment and position myself comfortably with a book or busy myself in the kitchen so that when he came in I could appear to be totally calm and unconcerned. These short excursions of his reassured him and helped to sustain his self-respect. I think they were crucial to his continuing cooperation and general good spirits. I regret, in retrospect, that I did not encourage him to take them more often.

A few evenings when I simply could not muster the energy to go out with him, Josh went out by himself for short walks in the neighborhood, never more than a few blocks. During one of these walks, he found on the book-rack of a liquor store a few blocks from the house a puzzle book called *Jumbles*. It was a series of words whose letters had been scrambled and which required rearranging to form proper words. He enjoyed this activity very much and with the passing of the months, as he became less capable of any physical activity, he would frequently spend several hours each evening lying on his bed, listening to music and working on these puzzles. When he had been through the whole book, we were not able to find any other similar collections, so I prepared sheets of jumbled words for him. Not only did he enjoy unscrambling them but he also felt it helped improve his ability to read.

Another quiet, sedentary activity that I initiated during the summer was card playing, which was important for him as an aid in number recognition as well as entertainment. In a short time he was able to handle the cards well, and while I originally permitted him to beat me at gin rummy, he was soon winning legitimately much of the time.

We tried to watch the political conventions on television during July and August but he found them confusing and preferred to discuss what was happening politically with me or with Leib. As the pre-election activities intensified he did try to follow the developments more closely and was looking forward to going to the polls in November.

And so, with these activities, the incredible number of

medical appointments we were constantly keeping, classes at the Fernald School, days at the beach, and whatever else I could think of for him to do, the summer passed.

Early in September we took Josh to Dr. Stark for the appointment we had set up concerning the chemotherapy. Dr. Stark described to him what the treatment would entail and what possible promise for improvement it held. Josh agreed to consider it and said he would call back in a day or two to let the doctor know his decision. He tried very hard during this particular visit to get Dr. Stark to tell him outright exactly what the prognosis was at this time for his future and the length of time he could anticipate. But the doctor did not seem to be willing to do this and avoided giving him a direct answer. When we left the office, Leib and I had to translate these evasions to Josh according to what the doctor had told us.

When we arrived home, I could see that Josh was depressed. I didn't realize how much so until we had occasion, after his death, to listen to the tape in which he discusses making the decision to end his life. Perhaps that might have been the wisest solution; I don't know. The fact is, though, that he decided against suicide at this time.


*Today is the 8th, September 8th, like I said. Yesterday (I go to the doctor once every four or five weeks) he looked again, then he went out, he left the room, he came back in and he had some bad news and I knew it, I knew it. The tumor is still growing. We have one hope left and we better think about that, they want me . . .*

*I — believe me, I'm not a fool, I'm not a fool. I've known for months. I'm not kidding myself, I know that I am just trying to appease* [sic] *the happiness that we are trying to have, to make life livable, to know what it's all about. We know what life means and what the opposite of life is all about—we may say—death. I knew I was not going to live. I know it now.*

*Yesterday, when I went to see the doctor, we talked about the treatment* [chemotherapy] *and I'll have it once and in another few weeks and then another time and then he talked about operating again.* *

*I don't like to use bad words but—bastard! Don't ever use that word on me! Nobody is cutting on my head again. Nobody will cut the parts of my head out.*

*I know that I'm dying. Why do they try to fool me? Even if you don't call it trickery or treachery we know this —I'm going to be dead soon and I have to accept it, which I have. I have accepted this for months. I have tried to prepare myself and I think that I have.*

*There are certain things to think about and talk about. I know that I will not have it any way but my way, which will be the right way, when it comes to . . . finishing things . . . shall I say. I'm trying to be a man. I want whoever hears this to not only think about it but to try to understand it— not reading it, not hearing it, not only feeling it but understanding it.*

*I know that it is going to be one of these treatments and then out, and then in and out, and that I'm getting worse. The only thing that's getting better on me is my reading and I should have normal reading for a person my age but with those tumors . . . I can't even read anymore. That's why I've been working at this . . . at this speech therapy. I have a wonderful teacher who is trying to help me, to try to help me get back to normal. But that is something that should already be there after you've already learned to read.*

*Well, lying here I think I know, I know what's going on. One day later, when you read this, please remember that,*

* At this point Josh misunderstood Dr. Stark. What the doctor said was that there would be no value to another operation; any further surgery would totally incapacitate him.

number one, I'm not a fool . . . and number two, I'm not afraid . . . number three, I'm not, the word is stupid. You know I'm still a heck of an intelligent person. I know what I know. My vocabulary and my speaking, of course, leaves much to be desired. I cannot talk as quickly as I used to, but as for my memory, it's all in my head. I know everything that I think and I feel. I'm just not quick with the wit, shall we say. So I will not have myself dragged to the very last piece of mediocrity and then torn apart and either have them say, or let them hear, that their son is dead or that he is a vegetable. I won't have it.

I hope very, very much that my body will not be buried. I do not like that at all. I wish for my body to be cremated. Abe Maslow [Josh's great-uncle] had his body cremated. People do die—we know that. Nobody's trying to evade the issue or anything like that. When a person dies they die and they know nothing about what's going on. You do not have to put a person's carcass down into a dirty hole and cover it up and put a few flowers on it and then try to imagine that you have a live person there. You don't. It's better, clean, proper and dignified to have a person and then the ashes thrown. The person will be remembered and it will be . . . accepted. I am not going to leave this area as a potato.

Anyway, I'm probably going to be lying down for a while now. Down, I am down now like you don't know, and down. But as for lying down, physically lying down, I think that — Now I have a really bad headache, a really bad headache. Boy-oh-boy, my head!

Please don't forget this, I want to make this perfectly clear [imitating President Nixon's voice]. I'm in complete control. I'm not a nut. I'm not sick, or drugged, or stoned with any kind of drug or anything like that. I'm not taking any drug except those which the doctor prescribes. Everything I say is the truth. Please believe me, Mom and Dad *and Simon. I'm quite aware of what is going on. I'm not going out of my mind, as you three are well aware. Someone else might not get the same things, might not read the same things, and might not understand everything. But you know, as well as I do, that I am a hundred percent sane. Sane—that doesn't mean that everything else is good. I don't mean that I've got a strong brain or something; I don't even have much of a brain left anyway, physically speaking, but I haven't lost my mind. I reckon that crazy people don't know that they have lost their minds. I'm sure there is no question in your minds that I'm a sane, rational person.*

*So much has been said this last bit of time. I hope you are not so thick, shall we say, as everything that I've said, is not pretty much out and out — it's all explained— what's going to happen.*

*I'm sure you realize this is all a recording now. It's hard for me to give it to you, and it's strange for you to believe it, and it's going to be so hard on you. You don't know how decimated I am about what's happened to two such beautiful people, my parents. And my brother. But we've gone through this many times in this recording. Death is death and that's it; you can't make up things about it.*

*Now, I don't think that you will think that I'm a horrible person. I've tried to explain what's going on. You know that I have to do this to myself—do it now.*

*Many months ago, when I was still in the hospital and Dad was saying—that's when I found out from the doctor that I was going to lose all my hair—this is a horrible thing for any young person to hear, it's enough to just drive you out of your mind. It's just terrible. You know all of your hair is going to be gone, you're going to have a big scar on your head. All I thought of was, please, I just wanted to— I couldn't really write yet or talk very well — but I remember that night. It was just horrible! I was pouring— I scratched* with a strong pen. "Kill me, kill me, please kill me!" But it never happened. Life was just kind of like a fresh breeze of air—although it might be dark outside or rainy. And that day went forever and I lived that day — and another day — and I knew that I would just have to accept all that crap. That's what I did . . . I was just juvenile. You know, you just have to do certain things.

What I have to tell you about now is not juvenile, and I'm not just being a crybaby, you all know that. You know what happened to me, you know why I have to do this. Let me say this one more time—if you don't get it clearly. My life is going, it is almost gone. They are going to try this or that, and hope for this or that, but in the end I'm dying and I'm going to be dead. I'd rather do it cleanly. I want to be in control. I will not have any missing pieces. It's going to be a nice clean thing—just zoom! I'm not going to just drag life out, ripping you poor people apart. Please don't think I'm foolish or crazy or don't know what's happening to me—or don't know how horrible this is going to be to you three, Mom, Dad and Simon. You'll have me on your mind for years. Of course you'll never forget me, but life will go on; my life will not go on. Please accept that it is not going on. It is dying. Your life is a regular life like most people's and you will— Life will go on.

It is hard for you people, but we've had a long happy time that we have spent. We've loved each other, so, so much. It's not like most families. I guess they all say this— those having had good families—but we love each other. We are smart, good people and we always want the best for the other, that's the truth. I am so happy and pleased, I am so fortunate and lucky, to have such fine parents. It is incredible that they are so concerned, and they are smart enough to be aware of it and try and do something about it. I also know that if they are honest to me, through me, for me, they will know that what I am doing, it's just a question of— It may not be this same day that this happens . . . Whether it happens now, or a week from now, soon enough it's going to happen. Before I have a real mess for myself, I'll do it this way.

I can't, I can't . . . I'm trying, I won't cry or anything like that. I don't think I'm doing that. I don't have much feeling left in my body, I mean in my heart, and the hard part of living, the hard part had already hit me when I was in the hospital. I wanted to die so badly, and it just wouldn't happen. I remember waking up the next day and I thought to myself, "Nothing is going to get me, nothing is going to make me cry anymore."

A little badness here and there, like when I went to the doctor the other day. I couldn't talk because I would have had to break. As long as I'm quiet I can control myself and my situation. But if I start talking, like yesterday when I left the doctor, I just can't talk. When my father wanted to talk to me, I just had to let it go, for just as soon as I start talking that would be it, I would just embarrass myself.

But believe me, I love everybody. I love them so, so much, so much, I mean it. I love you so much, you three are incredible. I wish, I wish I could be there, but please understand I still have that IQ. I still understand life so I'm not . . . I am not, in a sense then, I am not killing myself. I am recognizing myself. I understand myself and I am taking it like a man. I am.

Everybody, all my relatives have been so nice to me. Bubu and Zaida, Ruth, George and Edith, Babe and Anna, and all the other relatives—Ben Ami, Amnon and Marilyn, David, Zev—I hope I haven't forgotten . . . and Ima. Poor Aba, he is just a name. Everybody is just so nice. I love you so much.

It is extremely frightening to imagine all of a sudden being . . . Wow, that I do lose my mind and become nothing. That is beyond compare. That happened to me once *when I was in the hospital for about ten minutes, and I really thought I lost it all. But now, obviously, for all these months, I am in control. I love you so much. Please try to understand. Do not hate me for it. Please do not hate me for this. You know I'm not doing this out of meanness. It's anything but that.*

*I love you, and I love everybody. I do love the world, I really, really do. I've made an attempt, I've proven that I do. Everyone I talk to—I never, never downgrade anyone. I love everybody, I love you so much. Please don't forget me, please. IT'S JUST MY TIME. I know it's going to hurt you. I'm not horrible, you know all this. You'll just have to make do; you will. Things will be all right, I wouldn't want Dad to lose his job, or his work go bad, by doing this to him. But I've been waiting and waiting. This sickness is just driving me . . . I'm going to be dead.*

*Please, things will be all right, everything will be OK. You will remember me and that I was not a horrible person or anything like that. I love you so much. I do. Be good, everybody, please be good, please be good. I love you so much, I love you, I love you, I love you.*

Josh was most unenthusiastic about proceeding with the chemotherapy treatment. I tried throughout the course of Josh's illness never to impose my will on him. I knew that we shared a tremendous mutual admiration and respect. I also knew that his condition made him less able to dispute or disagree with me, and I did not want to force on him anything he did not want. But in this case, I did use a considerable degree of persuasion to convince him at least to try the chemotherapy. I knew he dreaded the thought of returning to the hospital. I knew he felt strongly that there was nothing ultimately to be gained. I knew he was convinced in advance that as with every procedure that had been tried, the negative side effects would be greater than any conceivable possible benefit. In spite of all this, and largely because Leib was determined that Josh should attempt this treatment, I was more energetic in my persuasion than my good sense dictated. I was wrong. I should not have imposed this additional physical burden on Josh. But I wanted my son to live. Although I knew he was not going to live, I tried to fool myself, to convince myself that this new physical torment would be helpful.

Josh reluctantly agreed that we should call the doctor and set up an appointment for his hospitalization. He was quite depressed at the thought of returning to the hospital. He knew that whatever progress he was making with his reading had reached a plateau and that there was no further advance in sight. His back was causing increasing difficulty. He had so little to look forward to. All he wanted was some peace, and we weren't even allowing him that.

At this time I got the idea of giving him a spectacular treat, something really exciting to look forward to. Next month, on October 10, Josh would be twenty-one years old. We decided that Leib would take Josh to Europe for three weeks to celebrate his birthday. I was sure this would be his last. Ever since our trip to Europe in 1965 he had spoken about returning to visit the people he knew, the places he had been. Before his illness, he had been planning just such a trip for this summer. Our financial circumstances were very strained and worsening rapidly. But this was good medicine, the best we could give him.

It was decided that I would not go with them, for several reasons—the first, of course, being monetary. There were two other considerations. I wanted Leib to have an opportunity to grow closer to his son while there was still a chance. Away from me, away from the house, away from the pressures of work, the constant financial concern, totally involved with each other for three weeks, they would have one last chance to learn more about each other, to become better friends. Finally, I was exhausted, and the opportunity for a few weeks by myself would give me a chance to rebuild my strength, to face whatever the future would bring and help me to help Josh through the time remaining to him.

We told Josh about our plans for his birthday, adding that we'd have to get the doctor's approval. I wrote to Dr. Stark and received a reply stating that he and his colleagues could see no reason why Josh should not take this trip; that, on the contrary, they thought it might be very good for his morale. Josh could hardly believe it. He became filled with excitement and we spent endless hours discussing the things he would do and see, the places they would visit, and the people they would meet again after all these years. For a brief time it became fun again for him to live. The promised trip to Europe may have been the one factor that decided him against ending his life at that time.

Josh was due to enter the hospital for his chemotherapy on September 20. Leib took him there in the morning, and I was shocked to find them back home again at about noon. Some procedural nonsense, a foul-up in the paperwork, had forced a postponement of his hospitalization for two weeks. Josh couldn't have been more disgusted. It had taken such tremendous energy and emotional output on his part to bring himself to the point of being willing to return to that hospital, which held such horrible memories for him. Now he would have to go through it all again in two weeks.

At any rate, the chemotherapy was delayed and Josh ended his summer bright with anticipation of his upcoming trip to Europe.

# Fall 1972

O God, forsake us not in time of trouble,
in days of distress. Help us endure . . .
Apocrypha, Ben Sira 36:1, 16

*You know, I was hoping that things would get better . . . I had a dream in my mind everything was going to get back to normal, back to beautiful—that life would be worth living. Every time I worked on myself to bring myself to that point and think that maybe I can take that thing — take that thing — I will, I will make it and everything like that, I'd get hit with another, another and another . . .*

There were so many things to do in preparation for the trip to Europe. Josh's and Leib's passports had expired, so they had to have new photos taken and renew their passports at the Federal Building. After careful shopping, we found a sheared sheepskin jacket for Josh that would be warm enough for the colder climate.

One of the big hurdles to be overcome was the renewal of Josh's driver's license (which expired on his birthday) so he could get an International Driver's License. Driving on the English country roads was one of the things he looked forward to most. He had always been fascinated by English cars and was particularly intrigued with the idea of driving on the left-hand side of the road. In fact, he told me repeatedly that because of the nature of his vision problem, he would actually be far more comfortable driving on that side.

We decided to resort to a bit of trickery in order to make sure that Josh would get the new license. We were not concerned about his knowledge of driving rules, but about the incredible strain on him of reading the test. Leib accompanied Josh to the Department of Motor Vehicles to take the test, and after making the application, Josh passed the test material to Leib, who filled out the answers. Josh then presented the test at the clerk's counter for checking. Of course, it all went off without a hitch, but when the two of them came home that day they were in a state of thorough nervous exhaustion. This behavior was so alien to both of them that they could not help feeling guilty.

Josh simply glowed with happy anticipation every evening as we discussed all the places they would go, whom they would see, and the interesting sights he would be able to film with his excellent new camera, for which he had bought two dozen rolls of film. The back pain that had been giving him so much trouble did not ease up, but his excitement and enthusiasm kept him going. Also, we increased his dosage of codeine to one and a half pills every three to four hours.

We finally settled on an itinerary that would start by direct flight to London, where they would stay for four or five days. The next five days would be spent touring the English countryside by rented car, and then they would fly to Amsterdam for a day, rent a car there and drive to Brussels, where so many of our old friends were. After a few days in Brussels, they would spend their remaining time in Paris, returning by direct flight from Paris to Los Angeles. The trip was to be for three weeks, the minimum time required for lower airfare rates; a shorter trip would have cost so much more in airfare that the difference would just about equal the added cost of staying longer in Europe.

We had a friend who was working on his doctoral dissertation at the London School of Economics, a young Canadian named Jeff whom we had met in 1964 when we lived in Brussels and with whom we had maintained an occasional correspondence through the years. At that time he was spending a year working abroad before entering the university. We had been quite friendly with him, had welcomed him to our home and through us he had met others of our friends. Leib wrote to Jeff about Josh's condition and what he would have to expect when he saw them again. He asked him to secure hotel accommodations in London and meet them at the airport.

Leib also wrote to our various friends in Brussels whom they were planning to see, again explaining in careful detail the facts about Josh's physical condition and handicaps. They must be ready to anticipate the limitations under which Leib and Josh would be functioning. We knew that our friends would be anxious to do many things to entertain them, to go places with them, but Leib told them to make no arrangements in advance. He explained that any activity that Josh found tiring would have to be forgone, and that his needs, his desires, and his interests would be paramount. In other words, anything Josh wanted, anything Josh felt comfortable with would take precedence over the normal amenities of visiting.

All the plans were shaping up well. Most of the important preparations such as securing passports, licenses and tickets and writing to our friends in Europe had already been taken care of by the time Josh entered the hospital on Tuesday, October 3, for the first chemotherapy treatment.

His hospital room was again on the sixth floor, in the same area where he had spent so many agonizing weeks during his first hospitalization. Many of the same staff personnel were still there. Josh remembered all of them by name and most of them remembered him well. He had been a patient there for so long that he felt more at ease than he had anticipated on returning to the hospital. Nevertheless, he was very reluctant to submit to the new treatment. He was doing it, I know, to please us, his parents.

The treatment itself, requiring as it did a few injections that lasted several hours each, was very taxing to his nerves and quite uncomfortable. Fortunately, his veins held up very well and there were no unfortunate side effects in the actual administering of the chemical. The only side effects he did suffer were slight nausea the first day, increased nausea the second day and vomiting on the third day, when he came home; but this reaction passed and did not recur. As had been promised, there was no mention made of an angiogram, but he did undergo more X rays and brain scans. He wasn't required during this hospitalization to be in bed or in pajamas, so he wore his street clothes during the day and only undressed at night to go to bed. I spent as much time each day with him as I could because he was bored and fretful and did not at all like being back in the hospital.

The same endless, repetitive questioning procedure to obtain his medical history was attempted again with Josh this time. Being in a different state of mind than he had been just after his operations, he struck back in small ways at what he considered to be taxing and irritating intrusions. All of the patients are subjected to this, particularly in a teaching hospital, and it is a real burden to the hospitalized person who is already suffering discomfort, apprehension and unpleasantness. I could thoroughly sympathize with Josh and, in fact, I even enjoyed some of the ploys and sly humor that he used.

One of the interns who came to the room to get a case history chose to question Josh just at lunchtime one day. I was there but did not participate; I just observed the exchange. Josh was sitting on the side of his bed with the lunch tray on the table before him. Hospital food is not terribly appetizing under the best of circumstances, but at least it was warm, having just been brought in, and Josh was hungry. It was at this particular moment that the intern chose to interrogate Josh. He positioned himself in front of Josh and started the routine questioning.

"Well, now, let's get some information about you. How are you feeling now?"

"I'm feeling hungry. I'd like to eat this stuff before it gets cold," Josh said, and then added "Why don't you come back later?"

The intern continued with the questioning. "What are your symptoms, what are your problems?"

Josh was nibbling at the food. "Undernourishment," he said under his breath.

"What? What did you say your problem is?" he repeated, busily fiddling with his clipboard.

"I can't see you," Josh stated loudly.

Very flustered, now, the intern asked with alarm, "Do you mean you are blind?"

"I mean what I said. I can't see you."

Clutching at straws, the doctor plunged on, "Are you here for surgery?"

Josh gently fingered the protruding flap on his semibald head. "Oh, man, you don't see me, either."

The intern couldn't seem to let go. Why, I wondered, doesn't the jerk just read the chart? Or look? Or listen? But he struggled on with a few more questions to which Josh answered with "Huh? What?"

By this time, the doctor finally got the message that Josh was putting him on and he left. I almost exploded with laughter. Later in the evening, when I came back to see him, I asked Josh if the doctor had returned to fill out the forms. Josh told me he hadn't.

There was another, even more foolish occurrence. A woman dressed in a white hospital jacket and carrying a clipboard came bouncing into the room, stopping first at the adjacent bed which was nearest the door, and blurted out with no explanation of what it was she was attempting to accomplish, "I'm doing a study in epidemiology and what are you in the hospital for?"

The man in the other bed said, "I'm here for an appendix operation."

She said, "Thank you!" and bounced over to Josh's bed. "I'm doing a study in epidemiology, what are you here for?"

He said, "I'm here for an appendix operation."

"Thank you," and she trotted out.

The next day she bounced back. There had been a change in patients, and a different man had been put in the first bed. This same silly woman popped in and announced to the man, "I'm doing research on epidemiology, what are you in the hospital for?"

"For a checkup on a urinary tract problem," he moaned.

Then she jogged over to Josh's bed again and said, "I'm doing a study on epidemiology, what are you here for?"

He said, "I'm here for some tests on a urinary tract problem."

She started to leave, but at the door it must have occurred to her that something strange was going on. She did a classical double take and then bounced off down the corridor. So much for the research that is done in this manner with hospital patients.

Dr. Burgholz, who was in charge of the chemotherapy program, saw Josh daily. I spoke with him at length about the back pains that Josh had been suffering and asked him if there was anything they could do to determine their cause and perhaps to relieve the pain. He told me, as Dr. Goldman had already suggested, that there was a possibility the cancer had seeded itself in Josh's lower back, but that they would try a new pain medication. We were given Percodan, which Josh took for a couple of days, but he found it less effective than the codeine, so he decided to stick with that. I also requested at this time that Josh be given a prescription for sleeping pills. Josh understood completely my purpose for securing that prescription. And we ordered month-long quantitities of all the medicines and drugs Josh was taking so he would have a more than adequate supply to take with him on his trip.

While Josh was in the hospital and Leib and I could converse freely at home, I tried to make him understand the degree of dysfunction caused by Josh's handicaps. This may seem strange, since Leib had been with us ever since Josh's return from the hospital, but the fact was that the only times he had ever been alone with Josh were the few occasions when they had gone together to see a movie. That had not required much activity on the part of Josh, or much conversation. Primarily, I wanted Leib to realize that the biggest single adjustment he would have to make would be to reorient his own time frame. Everything Josh did, from major activities through the most minor action or motion, would have to be estimated in advance, allowing at least double the normal time because he functioned in slow motion. Although Josh could now understand almost everything, even rather abstract and complex discussions, everything had to be presented to him in a simple manner and frequently restated so that he could follow the chain of thought. His personal care took an inordinate amount of time, and he was slow in making decisions. It was really a matter of readjusting one's entire time schedule to half the normal pace.

I also explained to Leib that although I had developed a seemingly easy manner with Josh, the reason Josh felt extremely comfortable with me was because I knew exactly the degree of his difficulty in understanding or speaking. When Josh and I were with other people, I frequently translated much of what was going on, in what had evolved

195

into a rather easy and quite inconspicuous way. But now Leib would be alone with Josh and it was important for him to prepare, in advance, great reserves of patience and an easy manner, so that his tension and concern would not be communicated to Josh.

I suggested that on the trip he try a schedule that would allow for sight-seeing or any other activity they chose: to start after breakfast but be back at the hotel by four o'clock at the latest, so that Josh could take a nap for an hour or two before dinner. They would then have the evening to do other things. Leib must understand that Josh had become totally unargumentative; arguing was simply too taxing for him. Therefore, when Josh was trying to express an idea or a preference, Leib should be extremely careful not to override it or be impatient while it was being explained to him. Otherwise, Josh, to avoid additional strain, would just agree to any suggestion Leib made whether he really wanted to or not.

Also, knowing our friends in Belgium, I warned him it was crucial to avoid what I was certain they would be planning—namely, large gatherings. Josh was not able to function comfortably in large groups with many voices, particularly in this case where there would be bilingual, or even trilingual, conversation all around him. Our friends might also attempt to arrange busy sight-seeing schedules, and Josh was not capable of maintaining a hurried pace. Since Josh was both unable and unwilling to enter into arguments, if Leib was not very protective of his needs and interests during their stay in Brussels, it could prove to be disastrous for Josh.

Leib listened carefully to everything I said. But he maintained layers of both psychological and intellectual reservations that I couldn't seem to peel away. He somehow couldn't quite accept the reality of Josh's diminished capacity—not Josh, not the son who had mirrored his own strong and handsome youth.

We were so fortunate to have Leib. How much we all leaned on him and how incredible his selfless acceptance of our dependency. He was fighting to maintain our family as his life disintegrated about him—a dying son, a lifetime's savings gone, a frightening and frustrating inability to earn an adequate income. Maybe he had to insulate himself with a subconscious refusal to admit how little Josh had left in order to sustain himself, his own capacity to function.

Josh came home from the hospital Thursday evening and that weekend we had some relatives over to wish him happy birthday and bon voyage. The following Wednesday, October 11, the day after Josh's twenty-first birthday, I drove them to the airport early in the afternoon and watched them board the plane. All went smoothly with the exception of one slightly uncomfortable circumstance. Because of the recent airplane hijackings, all luggage, including hand-carried bags, was carefully examined by guards before the passengers boarded the plane. One of the bags Leib was carrying onto the plane was a cosmetic case that contained Josh's huge array of medications. They were laid out with a schedule I had attached listing their quantities, times and frequency of use. Included were large quantities of dilantin, phenobarbitol, Decadron, codeine, Tretin-A, tetracycline, regular aspirin, seco-barbitol, and several jars of the antacid Josh had to take with each ingestion of medicine to reduce the nausea they caused. The guards immediately began to question Leib when they opened the case, but I spoke with Josh to distract his attention while Leib explained Josh's illness to the guards. Seeing that all the medications were from the UCLA pharmacy, the guards then passed Leib and Josh through with no trouble. They boarded the plane and I returned to the apartment.

Three whole weeks stretched before me without the constant responsibility and emotional exhaustion of caring for my son, worrying about his every need, agonizing with him through his pain. I thought it would be easy to relax, unwind, refresh my dwindling stores of energy so that I would be ready to resume these burdens and responsibilities when Josh returned. I hoped they would have a wonderful time. There was no reason to anticipate any dramatic new physical problems with Josh, and Leib was prepared to handle anything that might arise. The problem I had constantly feared, that Josh might suffer a seizure, was terrifying to me because of the disparity in our sizes, but Leib at six feet five inches and two hundred and twenty pounds was more than a match for Josh. They had ample supplies of medication and should the unforeseen happen, they were after all going to be in civilized countries with adequate medical attention available.

In anticipation of this time when I would be alone, numerous friends and relatives had arranged dinner or luncheon engagements with me. I had tried to explain to them that, although I did want to see them under circumstances that would permit me to be more myself, more relaxed without attending to Josh's needs, I really needed some time by myself, if for no other reason than just to be able to sleep undisturbed.

That first evening, I had promised to dine with my friend Charlotte. The evening alone with her was in a sense representative of many of the evenings I would have with other friends and relatives. Subjects that had not been discussed before we were now able to speak of freely without the constraint of my immediate concern for Josh or the knowledge that he was nearby and could perhaps overhear. It was interesting that with each person the discussion brought up some different aspect or question about Josh's illness, the relationship between Josh and myself and thoughts about life and death.

Charlotte suggested that this devastating illness must be

more difficult, more disastrous for Josh than it would be for some other young man, in view of the fact that he had been so superior in every way. For him to suffer these multiple disfigurements, incapacities, and dysfunctions might be more traumatic, starting as he did from so high a plane. She said, "Mash, maybe this is your fault. You always expected so much from him. And he always lived up to the expectations. Even the way you looked at him . . . how could he help but know he was beautiful?"

This thought had never occurred to me. I remember answering rather defensively, "Oh, come on, Charlotte. That isn't quite fair. What's wrong with supporting a child in his self-confidence? Sure Josh has a well-developed ego, but why shouldn't he? He isn't immodest; he just knows what he has . . . or had."

"But he knew he was special," she continued.

"Dammit. What was I supposed to do? Prepare him to die at twenty-one without it mattering?"

The conversation turned to other subjects. But that thought was to keep recurring to haunt me for the rest of Josh's life. Had I done him a disservice? Was it harder for him because he had been so exceptional? After his death, it was a genuine solace to me to hear Josh refer to this very subject in the first of his tapes. He attributes part of the strength he demonstrated throughout his illness to this sense of confidence and appreciation of his own worth. And he expresses his gratitude to me and to his father for having instilled in him the belief in his own abilities.

With another friend, the subject of God came up. She told me, "I've been giving a lot of thought to this since Josh's illness. In rather a vague way, I've always thought that there must be some sort of Supreme Being that directs the destiny of men. Do you feel that maybe there is some grand pattern, some purpose in this illness?"

"I've never believed in God, Phyllis. At least not what I

think you're talking about. A personal God that directly controls individual lives?"

"Yes. That's what I meant. Can Josh's sickness have a bigger meaning?" she questioned me.

"What meaning? A pointless destruction. If I had believed in God before Josh got sick, I sure as hell wouldn't now. Why Josh? Because he's always been good? Bright? Handsome? What kind of irrational 'pattern' or 'plan' would that be?" I was furious.

She persisted, "But maybe there is a meaning for the future . . . something we don't know about."

"Sure, for the future. That's why he's dying now, before he even had a child." How I had dreamed since his operation of his leaving a child—a baby, a new Josh. It would have been more bearable then. I'd fantasized about Julie coming back and saying she was pregnant by him and she wanted us to take the baby. "There isn't any reason to this. It's a random accident of nature. What kind of stupid God would do this?"

Late Sunday night I put through a call to their hotel in London; allowing for the time difference, it was about nine o'clock Monday morning. Leib answered, and we had a short talk; I couldn't speak with Josh since he wasn't awake yet; Leib assured me that everything was going well, that Josh felt, if anything, better there than he had at home and that they were really enjoying themselves. They had mailed cards which should be arriving soon. There was something in Leib's voice that didn't reassure me although he insisted everything was fine. What nonsense, I told myself—just inventing trouble.

After that, I received a postcard daily from either Leib or Josh, and frequently from both. As I eagerly read the cards from Josh, I analyzed them for clues as to how he was feeling. It seemed to me, with the arrival of each new postcard, that there was some sort of decline in his happiness and excitement. The cards were consistently pleasant, and I told myself it was just possible that I was reading into them things that simply were not there. I would interpret two or three misspellings as tension on his part. In several cards he mentioned how much he missed me, and I thought this might mean he wasn't comfortable with Leib. Still, all the cards sounded happy, and they were arriving with great regularity so that I was able to follow the course of the trip.

I received one letter from Leib which he wrote while Josh was asleep one day. In it he said, among other things, "I now know more fully, I now more fully comprehend what you meant by Josh's limitations and I know how difficult it has been for you these past months." I confess it was an extremely selfish thought on my part, but when that letter arrived, for the first time since Josh had come home from the hospital, I felt that someone else truly understood what it had been like, caring for Josh for all those months. I was no longer so completely alone with my hideous visions of what Josh had yet to face.

The second Saturday after they left for Europe I arranged to spend with Simon. In a way, I knew I was being most unfair to him, but all of my energies and concerns were so totally involved with Josh that it was difficult for me to look upon Simon as the individual he was, rather than as the brother of Joshua. I felt that being alone with him, it might be possible to make some new contact with my younger son. I wanted him to do more for Josh; but whether or not he did, he was still my boy and would soon be my only child.

I went to San Diego in the morning. Simon was waiting for me and seemed genuinely pleased that I had come. His room was well organized, he was neatly groomed and dressed, his schoolbooks were on his desk, everything seemed very proper and orderly. Shortly after I arrived he offered me a cup of coffee, and wandering into the kitchen after him, I could not help but notice that the refrigerator was virtually bare. He was now on a very minimal budget, as we had reduced our allowance to him, but this was worse than I had anticipated. After our coffee we went to the local market where I purchased what I thought would be enough groceries to last him for at least several weeks to come. We came back to the house, loaded up the refrigerator and settled down for a talk.

We spoke for quite a while about Josh. Simon told me that he tried in his way to do what he could for Josh but he really felt he could not give more of himself. He found it terribly difficult to spend time with Josh. He was distressed by his handicaps and couldn't find a comfortable level for conversation. He would try harder after Josh returned from Europe, but he simply didn't think there was much more he could do. He told me something rather bittersweet at this time; it was so insightful of himself, but there was still some barrier he had within himself that made him incapable of altering the situation. He said, "Mom, you know whatever it is I finally do with my life, I'd better be very successful, because I'm gonna have to have a helluva lot of money to pay for the psychiatrist to help me get rid of all the guilt I'm building up now." After that, there was no benefit to be derived from my belaboring the point. He was incapable then, for whatever reasons, of giving more to Josh.* Like his brother, he was a realist. Should I then be less of one?

We spent a good afternoon together. He drove me over to the campus and we walked around a little. Then we

* Since I first wrote this there have been several in-depth studies done on public television about attitudes among the young toward death and the dying. In many cases youngsters are totally unable to even speak with, let alone, see the terminally ill sibling. Simon was just eighteen.

went to a nearby shopping mall and I bought him a few sweaters and a jacket because the weather was starting to turn cool. We really had been almost overlooking Simon— no food, inadequate clothing. How else were we failing him?

We had dinner together at an Italian restaurant and then I returned to Santa Monica. The visit had made us feel perhaps a bit more comfortable with each other, a little less angry than before. There was still something, some indefinable quality missing in our relationship. We were still just defending our different positions rather than helping each other. I simply didn't know what else to do to remedy that situation. It was all so unfair—to Josh, to Simon, to Leib and to me!

I had dinner with Marilyn and Amnon one evening. Marilyn teaches nursing at one of the state universities and she had taken her training at UCLA. We talked in considerable detail about Josh's physical problems and more or less reviewed the whole course of his illness. She offered the only explanation that ever made sense, however distorted, of the incredible errors that contributed to his second operation. "Dr. Stark wasn't there, his colleague was ill, so Josh was left in the care of the residents. You just don't understand the awe in which Dr. Stark is held at UCLA. When I was there, everyone practically stood at attention when he walked by. The residents were so paralyzed with fear that they might do something wrong with his patient that they were simply incapable of doing anything until the situation became critical." If she was correct, what irony! Because we had the best surgeon, Josh had the worst postoperative care.

I saw some other friends, visited with my folks, spent a few days lazing around the apartment. I devoted one day to shopping for a new outfit to please Josh on his return. The days were long and lonely but the weeks were speeding by. And so the time passed. Josh was never out of my thoughts for more than a moment or two. I was not uncomfortable with this sensation, but Josh's absence didn't give me complete relief from strain and worry because I was almost more concerned knowing I was not there should he need me.

About four or five days before they were due back from Europe, I received a visitor late one evening—Edwin, the son of one of our Belgian friends who had been traveling throughout Canada and the United States. His visit was not totally unexpected, but I had not known exactly when he would be arriving. We had hoped he would come before they left for Europe so that Josh would have an opportunity to see him. Edwin was just slightly older than Josh and they had been fairly good friends during the time we lived in Brussels. Since he had not arrived before their departure, I had hoped he would not come until the men had returned from Europe, but there he was, late one evening, dirty and hungry. Of course I welcomed him; under normal circumstances, it would have been such a pleasure to see him.

Edwin had developed into an unusual young man, quite interesting and very mature for his age. He had traveled widely in Europe, Africa, India, and Afghanistan and was now spending some months in Canada and the United States. When we had known him in Europe, he did not speak English, but in the intervening years in school, at the university and in his travels, he had learned English, so I was not forced to rely on my limited and inadequate French. The last few days of October before Josh and Leib returned, I was busy attempting to entertain this young man as best I could. I took him to see some of the sights in the area, and I drove down to San Diego one day so that he could visit with Simon. The time passed very quickly with Edwin there until it was Thursday, November 2, and I had to go and meet my family at the airport.

With a demonstration of the maturity he had developed, Edwin suggested that perhaps I wished to go alone. And indeed I did. I was concerned, apprehensive and nervous. I knew Josh would be very tired after the long flight back, and of course I had my premonitions that things were not going as well as they seemed. I dressed in the new outfit I had bought for the occasion and drove to the airport to meet the five-forty afternoon flight from Paris.

The plane arrived exactly on time. I watched the huge aircraft touch down as gently and softly as a glider in the gathering dusk and taxi to the unloading zone. As the passengers got off, I saw Leib and Josh. They were searching the crowd with their eyes. Suddenly, Josh spotted me waving from the crowd and I could see his face break into a great smile. As I had suggested, Josh had bought a wild hat in England—he had picked a checkered deerstalker— and he was wearing a new turtleneck sweater and his sheepskin coat. But smile and outfit could not disguise his condition. I was shocked by his appearance; he looked so dreadfully pale, so pitifully thin and weak. He waved to me as they walked down the steps from the plane. After that I waited for a long time as passengers and luggage went through customs inspection. They were on a 747 and it apparently had been carrying a full passenger load. Finally, after about an hour, they were cleared through customs and came out to meet me.

We were just delighted to see each other, Josh and I. "Hey, old lady, you know something funny? I really missed you!"

"That's okay. I can tell you something even weirder than that. I actually missed having you around the place bugging me, you cockamamie kid. Say, that's some great chapeau, beau."

"Yeah, I got it in London, first thing. You look good, Mom. That's a nice suit."

"I'll bet you're both tired after that long flight. Let's get home."

Indeed Josh was very tired and his walking, I could see, was extremely strained. He was in considerable pain.

On the ride back to the apartment he started telling me all about the trip and the places they had been, but I could see that as much as he attempted to make it sound marvelous, he had real reservations about the way the trip had gone. Leib was also telling me about the trip. I noticed that every time Leib started to speak, Josh would immediately become silent, so I asked Leib to please let Josh talk. I gathered from this small interchange that the three weeks had not really been long enough, contrary to what Leib indicated in his letter, for him to learn fully how to permit Josh the time to express his wants, his interests and his thoughts. I thought, "Damn it! Couldn't anything go well for my beloved Josh?"

I told them that Edwin was waiting at the apartment and Josh seemed pleased about that. As soon as we got home and Josh got his warm outer clothing off, I started to prepare something to eat while the fellows chatted in the living room. We no sooner sat down at the table than I could see Josh was having difficulties. He walked to his room to lie down and I followed immediately after. He was having a reaction that he had had occasionally before. This problem would occur at times of great stress or excitement or exhaustion: Not a seizure but rather a vagueness overcame him, a weakness, and he would speak in strange combinations of words, unable to say anything clearly or in logical order. We had found from past experience that the best way to handle this was for him to lie down while I sat beside him on his bed and held his hand tightly. Very quietly and very slowly I reassured him, told him that everything was all right, that he was fine, that this would pass in a moment. He lay there mumbling sounds and looking at me with those beautiful, large, liquid eyes, so filled with fear, a frightened, concerned hart—dear heart. All I could do was hold his hand, tell him it would be all right, tell him how much I loved him. In a short while it passed and he was well again and able to speak. He was so very tired. I insisted that we defer any further talking till the next day and he undressed and got into his pajamas, I gave him his medicines, and he went to sleep. My sweet son, my sweet damaged boy was home again.

Friday morning I was able to assess Josh's condition with greater accuracy. We talked about the trip. Josh was relaxed now and not too uncomfortable but there had been new developments. His stomach had been giving him trouble. First he had diarrhea on the trip and now he was constipated. This was a serious matter in his case and something Dr. Stark had repeatedly warned us to guard against. We immediately got milk of magnesia for him and with that, the food at home, and the routine re-established, within a day or two his stomach problems cleared up. But he was getting headaches more frequently. His back had given him some difficulty initially on the trip, and as time passed, it had reached extreme proportions. Now he could barely move around at all. Every step was an agony and the codeine was not strong enough to provide adequate relief. He was only comfortable lying down.

Josh was certain that the deterioration in his back condition was directly traceable to the chemotherapy he had undergone. He said that at the time the BCNU was administered he had felt it burning throughout his veins. He felt that the degree of deterioration, the rapidity with which the pains had increased following this treatment and the severe headaches all suggested a correlation. I agreed with him that the timing could indicate a relationship.

However, we had been given no warning to expect any of these side effects. It could be just a coincidence. I promised Josh that I would take steps as rapidly as possible to get some relief for him from these excruciating backaches.

Edwin proved to be excellent company for Josh. He also was very interested in classical music, and they had other interests in common to talk about, besides bringing each other up to date on what they had done during the past several years. Apparently Edwin found it easy to converse with Josh, and they had a very enjoyable visit throughout Friday and part of Saturday. Edwin left Saturday afternoon to go up north for a week to San Francisco to visit some people he had met. He promised to stop back to see us once again before returning to the East Coast and from there home to Europe.

Saturday my parents came to visit Josh and Sunday some other relatives came to see him. He was gradually feeling better, and he spoke more about the trip, much of which had been very good indeed. He loved England and had enjoyed the entire stay there, both in London and traveling through the countryside. The only really sour note had been that Leib only let Josh drive a few miles; he had been so obviously nervous and uncomfortable that Josh just turned the wheel back to him.

One of the real highlights of his trip had occurred in Brussels. Roger, a friend who worked for the Citroën people there, took Josh for an absolutely mad night ride through Brussels in one of the magnificent Citroën SM sports cars that Josh so admired every time we passed them in the showroom on Wilshire Boulevard. It was a memorable evening for him.

But the pleasure of the trip had begun to diminish when they got to the Continent. Josh was not feeling as well there and, as I feared, there were too many people trying too hard to insist on activities that he found difficult or uninteresting. Paris, where they spent the last five days of their trip, was only so-so. Leib and Josh felt that the city had deteriorated tremendously since we had last seen it. Smog was pervasive, prices were outrageous and, unfortunately, the French had not become any more pleasant or polite to Americans. By then Josh was eager to get home.

He had used all the film he had taken with him and had even bought a few more rolls in Europe. Josh assured me that some of the footage would be spectacular.

But when we got the film back from being developed and he ran through it for us, he was quite disappointed. There was far more repetition, and long stretches with little movement, than he had been aware of during the actual filming. Still, some portions were very interesting indeed, and he had gotten some quite unusual shots. He decided to do some drastic editing, cutting out portions that seemed repetitious or uninteresting to him or were in some way technically not as good as he would have liked. He worked at it intermittently but never did finish editing them completely. The strain of sitting up and concentrating was frequently too much for him; also as time passed, I think he simply lost interest.

All in all, although there had been some disappointments in the trip, Josh was very pleased to have had the opportunity to go. Now that he was home and some of his physical problems were being attended to, his spirits were reviving. With the passing of his tiredness and the other discomforts, in retrospect the trip grew in pleasure.

The next Monday we started back on the old routine. His first visit was to Dr. Marie. He couldn't wait to see her because his acne, reasonably well-controlled during the summer, had become exacerbated during the trip, perhaps as a result of the change of diet or water or climate. His face was bad, but his torso was unbelievable. When I took him to the doctor's office he wanted me to come in during his treatment period. (After his return from Europe, he wanted me with him during all treatments and examinations, and we became even more inseparable than before.) He had huge suppurating sores on his chest and back, some as wide as an inch in diameter and oozing blood and pus. The sores were painful and irritating, and his whole body felt sticky. Dr. Marie did a magnificent job working on him, cleaning him up. Gradually after that, with continued treatments, we were able to improve the condition. However, these new eruptions left his body badly scarred.

The next morning, I took him to an osteopathic physician with whom I had made an appointment when I realized just how painful his back had become. This doctor had been highly recommended to us and I thought his massaging technique might provide some relief for Josh's back condition. I gave him a detailed account of Josh's medical history and, perhaps as a result of that, he was so tentative in his application of massage that there was no benefit derived from our visit there. In the afternoon we went to the Fernald School and Josh had a great reunion with Barbara, his teacher. He had really missed her, and I think she had missed him as well.

We saw Dr. Goldman on Thursday. It was the usual unproductive visit. After an office wait of close to an hour (although we had an appointment), we had perhaps five minutes with him in the examination room, interrupted half a dozen times by telephone calls. He could provide no new suggestions for the pain Josh was suffering, but I did secure a prescription for more codeine.* Those visits were so frustrating, and one felt so helpless, so dependent on the doctors for the prescriptions. We were—as are all the sick in our country—suppliants, and as such waited endless hours for the crumbs of time indifferently dispensed. I

* A prescription for codeine, as a narcotic, is not refillable.

struck back in the one way I could without hurting Josh. Since Dr. Goldman was the only doctor we saw who was really disturbed by the Medical arrangement, I saved our stickers for him. Since we only had two a month, I had to pay for most office visits by personal check and could easily have used the chits elsewhere and paid Dr. Goldman directly. Maybe this sounds petty, but the weak fight with whatever weapons are at hand.

About this time, Edwin came back to visit us for another day or two before leaving for the East Coast. He promised to send Josh some European recordings of Beethoven symphonies, and Josh in turn promised to send Edwin some American recordings of Kentucky Bluegrass music, primarily banjo music, which appealed to Edwin very much. After Edwin left, I thought how unfortunate it was that he was not located permanently in this area. He had demonstrated an ability to communicate comfortably with Josh that none of Josh's other young friends had been able to manage. I think this was partly a reflection of the maturity these two young men shared—Edwin as a result of his travels and wider experience of the world and Josh because of his illness. They also shared a mutual disenchantment and disappointment with other young people of their age.

Josh was due to enter the hospital the following week for the second chemotherapy treatment. He just didn't want to go. He was convinced that not only had the first treatment done him no good but that it had created greater problems for him in various ways. Now he told me that, in addition to the sharp increase in the level and frequency of back pain he suffered, on two occasions while in Europe he had experienced tremendous cracking sensations within his brain. He said it felt like a melon being smashed open —that there was no other way to explain it other than a snap and a cracking sensation. I was inclined to agree with

Josh that if he didn't want the treatment and felt so strongly that it just caused more problems, he shouldn't be pushed. On the other hand, the doctors had never suggested any such side effects and I still couldn't slough off almost half a century of indoctrination about the infallibility of doctors. Leib was still very much in favor of his continuing the three treatments which supposedly would indicate whether or not the chemotherapy would benefit Josh.

I called Dr. Burgholz and told him that Josh felt there was a relationship between the chemotherapy and the new sensation he had felt in his brain and the increased back pain. Dr. Burgholz told me there was no reason to believe there was any causative basis in the treatment for Josh's decline. I relayed this to Josh and convinced him to return for the second treatment. I should not have done it; it was unfair. It was exactly what I had tried so hard to avoid throughout Josh's illness, this imposition of my wishes and attitudes on him. He really did know best what was happening inside him. Nobody, not even the doctors, were ever as aware of the development of his malignancy as he was.

On November 15 he went back to the hospital for the second treatment. On the second day, Josh freaked out. I have no other way to describe what happened; it was exactly like the descriptions one reads of a bummer, a bad acid trip. Something in the chemical had caused a strange and frightening upset in his brain. He hallucinated and screamed in terror. In all the months of Josh's illness, in spite of the strains and stresses he had undergone, he had always maintained absolute control over his reactions, over his mind and body. Now, for the first time, he was temporarily out of control. The doctors administered tranquilizers to him, and in time the reaction passed. We halted further treatment and took him home. Thereafter, along with the other medications Josh was required to take we had to add Valium for those occasions when these hallucinations and sensations of fear and disorientation would come upon him, which they did periodically and apparently randomly, with no discernible pattern. I wonder whether Josh was the only patient to suffer this reaction to BCNU.

*We knew that the tumor was still growing and we had to get rid of it. So we tried cobalt. It took about another six weeks. It's another way, the cobalt, to kill the tumor. That didn't work. We tried that, and we tried other things. We tried chemotherapy and that didn't work either. It only made things worse. It really made my head hurt.*

*I was in severe pain, and my back was just getting out of hand. My back had just been — going from worse to worse. The pain has just gotten worse and worse. You know, we started out with one pill maybe once or twice a day; I got to the point of two every day. Now I'm at the point where I have to take more and more and more and more—louder, louder, louder. Anyway, this pain's just gotten out of hand.*

*For my twenty-first birthday, you know, it was a gift, my father and I decided we were going to go to Europe and we went—for three weeks. We left on October 11th and we came back just after three weeks — in three weeks more we were back. I guess it was right at the beginning of November. Man that pain—whoooo, it just got me! I just couldn't move. Every morning I would take over an hour before I could get up. I could hardly walk. I couldn't do very much and it wasn't the happiest thing.*

*That was right after we went for the chemotherapy. We went for that and, oh, God! It made the pain so much worse. It really ruined things. All I can say is we went for that, and we tried that again (you have to wait for six weeks before you go again; it drains your blood) — It didn't do it. That pain!*

*Let's see, what did we do? You see my talking gets a little bit mixed up. What did happen—what did happen? We tried to get rid of that pain. We don't know what it is, what it did, what it does, and what it's for, and a lot of other words like that.*

While Josh was in the hospital, we saw Dr. Stark as well as Dr. Burgholz. The intensity of the back pain, in light of his case history, indicated now that there must be a malignancy in his lower spine. Dr. Stark said they could perform a spinal tap, a mylogram, to confirm this. But it would be unpleasant and possibly dangerous to Josh, and there would be nothing they could do anyway other than to confirm what we already knew. We would just have to treat the pain as best we could.

The medication Josh was taking for pain no longer seemed to be doing the job. I felt that since all the doctors seemed to offer was ever greater doses of narcotics, perhaps acupuncture would be an effective alternative. Dr. Stark was totally unreceptive to this idea. He suggested that Josh take to his bed for at least a week, moving only to go to the bathroom and not getting up for any other activity; even his meals should be served to him lying down. This seemed to me a very negative response. I told Dr. Stark that in my view, Josh was living under sufficiently limited conditions of activity as it was. The few things that gave him some sense of participation in the world, such as his classes at Fernald, were very important to him, and I couldn't see imposing this awful restriction on him in the vague hope that it might be beneficial. We left it pretty much at that—unresolved, and with both of us a bit angry.

When Josh got home he was so uncomfortable from the back pain and so depressed after the violent reaction to the chemical that in fact he did stay in bed for three or four days, but with not quite all the restrictions Dr. Stark had suggested. He felt fairly comfortable lying down, though there seemed to be no improvement in his condition if he moved.

I knew they had initiated an extensive program of testing acupuncture techniques at White Memorial Hospital. I called them and was told there was a six-month waiting period before they would accept any new patients. I explained there was a strong likelihood my son would not survive for six more months. They were very sorry but they said that most of the people who contacted them were in situations as desperate as ours, and all they could do was to put us on the waiting list. My last hope was Dr. Stark. I telephoned him and insisted that we wanted to try acupuncture as an analgesic; surely he could put us in touch with someone who practiced this technique. Reluctantly he gave me the name of a Dr. Levitz in the anesthesiology department of UCLA, who was experimenting with the procedure. I called Dr. Levitz and explained the situation, and we set up an appointment for the afternoon of December 1.

Not only walking but even sitting upright was now painful for Josh. He frequently spent the evenings in his bedroom lying down. We decided to purchase a reclining armchair for him so he could maintain an almost horizontal position and still be with us in the evening in the living room, perhaps watch television or talk with us or listen to music. We found a comfortable recliner for him in a store nearby in Santa Monica and, to avoid waiting the usual week for delivery, arranged for Leib to pick it up with the help of the son of the apartment manager. When they brought the armchair to the apartment, Josh and I

215

were waiting for them. They were having great difficulty at the entrance and could not seem to get it through the narrow hallway into the living room. Josh quietly watched them struggle for a few moments. Then he suggested that since it was a recliner, if they simply put it into a horizontal position, they would be able to bring it in with no trouble at all, which they did, and very soon it was set up in the living room for him.

This was only one demonstration of Josh's grasp of logic, which never diminished at a time when his other abilities seemed to be declining or to have reached a plateau. A similar incident also occurred at about this time. Josh and I had gone down to the basement garage to get our car one day, and there was a young man there who had just loaded his Volkswagen van in preparation for leaving. He, his father, his girlfriend, and several other people were upset because the van, loaded with bundles on the roof rack, couldn't clear the overhang and it seemed they wouldn't be able to drive it out of the garage. Josh sized up the situation immediately and, very sweetly, he suggested that if they just let a little air out of the tires, the vehicle would clear with no problem. We watched while they did it and, sure enough, the young man was able to pull out with no difficulty.

It was about this time that Josh decided to sell his car. It had been something of a burden to us during all these months; not only was there the expense of maintenance and insurance, but there was also the problem of parking it. We had no additional space in the garage and so had to move it on the street constantly and had occasionally gotten parking tickets. Josh had not wanted to give it up, hoping that perhaps things would get better and he would be able to use it more frequently. Now it was apparent to him that he would never be using the car again.

Josh had sold the other cars he had had since he was sixteen and had found it rather easy to do. We placed an ad in the local paper, but he insisted on handling the sale himself. He spoke to the callers on the telephone and when the first customer came he went alone with him to the garage. A short while later he returned, smiling broadly and clutching a handful of bills. "Look at that bread! I sold it for full asking price. How about that!"

"Josh, I've always told you you'd have a great future as a used car salesman."

"Well at least *we* know what the world is losing."

He now had a few hundred dollars at his disposal, and we no longer had the burden of worrying about the vehicle. I assured him, of course, that any time he wanted my car for his use, it was available to him.

Josh's decision to sell his car was another demonstration to us that he completely accepted the fact that his condition was not going to improve. In giving up the symbol of his independence and of a future, he was telling us that he was making this accommodation and was hoping, I think, that we would too.

At school, it seemed that his reading ability had slipped somewhat from its highest point, and although it now restabilized there was no further improvement. He was participating more in word games than he had before, since his physical activities were so much more limited. He played for hours with the Jumble games, and we also started playing Scrabble together. He was, as with everything he did, very slow, but on those days when he was not in too much pain and was able to sit up for several hours at a time, he played a remarkably good game and seemed to enjoy the challenge.

On Thanksgiving, Simon came home for the day and we sat down to a family dinner at the apartment. The brothers had a nice quiet visit. Josh talked to Simon about various things, and tried to get him to understand many of the attitudes he had been developing about a more mature approach to life and not wasting his youth on stupid habits that would cause him problems in the future. It was calm and peaceful, and they seemed genuinely to enjoy being with each other.

On November 30 a small article appeared in the *Los Angeles Times* about a remarkable recovery from a glioblastoma (closely related to Josh's tumor) by a young European man after treatment at the Tokyo University Hospital. Several friends called to tell me about it. The article described in general terms a different radiation technique from the one Josh had undergone. Leib immediately contacted Dr. Timmons at the radiation department of UCLA and asked him about this treatment. Dr. Timmons was aware of the procedure and said it required a modified nuclear reactor that emits slow neutrons. A nonradioactive isotope (Boron II) is injected into the patient and surrounds the malignant tumor; bombardment of Boron II isotope with slow neutrons causes secondary radiation to be emitted by the isotope, which then directly affects the malignant cells and seemingly does not damage healthy cells. Therefore, far greater radiation levels can be used to destroy the malignant cells. Dr. Timmons referred to this as "a tremendously exciting technique." He had been aware of it for several years but had been unable to obtain a grant, or other funding of the $500,000 needed to modify UCLA's reactor, finance a research program for chemists and neurologists, and run a number of empirical research tests to determine the dosage of Boron II and radiation required. He was very discouraged that the required funding was not available because of the "exciting possibilities" which could result from such a research program.

It was incredible! The richest country in the world, which didn't hesitate to spend a million dollars to kill each of the North Vietnamese we'd been slaughtering for eight years, couldn't make available funds to institute a program of this type.

Our next thought was whether we could borrow the money to take Josh to Japan. I tentatively broached the subject of a new treatment to Josh, and it was the only time he got furious with me since his hospitalization. "Don't you undertsand all I've been telling you for months?" he shouted. Then quietly, "I am thoroughly ruined inside. I am an old, old man; all worn out. There is nothing left to save." Then he restated all his losses, he reminded me that the cancer was also in his back, and he said what I had thought so many times myself. "I never recovered from surgery, Mom. You know that. The swelling never went down after they took out part of the tumor. There should have been less pressure then for a while, but there was more. Some other damage was done. It's not just the tumor—it's everything. I'm all used up." We never discussed it again.

Finally, it was December and time for the first acupuncture treatment. We met Dr. Levitz in a treatment room in the hosipital. A short, young Jewish doctor, he came in with a Chinese-American intern, both dressed in unironed green surgery outfits including caps and shoe covers. He spoke with us about Josh's condition and explained the treatment to us. He had a cheap cardboard box with Chinese lettering containing long, metal pins which would be inserted at specific points in Josh's body to treat the back pains. Some of them he would hook up to the very low voltage battery that would vibrate them, others he would spin or vibrate by hand periodically. He assured Josh that the treatment was not painful and that it did frequently have favorable analgesic results. We told him we understood; we had no idea of utilizing this as a cure for anything, but if it could in some way help Josh's pain, that was all we were hoping for from the treatment.

I asked him how much experience he had had with acupuncture and what the results had been. He told me he had studied with a Korean acupuncture specialist for about a year but that shortly before this time (it was still illegal to use acupuncture in the United States) the Korean man with whom he had been studying had had to go underground to avoid prosecution. He was now continuing to study on his own. The young Chinese-American intern who was with him knew nothing about acupuncture but had some limited ability in reading Chinese and was helping to do research from the Chinese texts; he in turn was teaching the intern what he had already learned about the placement of the needles.

If Josh's condition hadn't been so serious, this would have been hysterically funny. What a combination! The little Jewish doctor with big needles, the Chinese-American intern witnessing acupuncture for the first time and, somewhere, a Korean expert hiding from the police—and as background to this black comedy, the reluctance of most of our medical wizards to accept the witchcraft of another society.

After changing into a hospital gown, Josh was made to lie face down on a bed. The doctor inserted numerous pins in his lower back, one or two in the upper back and quite a few in his ankles. There is no explanation yet as to *how* acupuncture works, but there is considerable documentation that it *does* work.* The doctor could not explain why the pins are put in the ankles, for instance. But the fact is that these are methods that have been employed for hundreds of years and, in fortunate cases and under expert handling, do work.

The entire procedure took no more than half an hour. While Josh was dressing, the doctor spoke with me again;

* Since Josh's experience with acupuncture, there has been a great deal more testing of the technique in the U.S. Recently the newspapers carried an article describing its use as the sole anesthetic in a Caesarian birth.

he said that he himself had such limited knowledge, but he had had some success in treating back pain in other patients and was hopeful that he could help Josh. Josh was to come three times in weekly intervals, and by the end of the third treatment we would be able to gauge the effects of the treatment.

Afterwards, Josh and I went into Westwood and stopped for coffee at an outdoor cafe. He assured me that the treatment had not been uncomfortable or painful. He didn't feel any improvement, but the doctor said that was not to be expected this soon and he was hopeful that perhaps a few more treatments would produce beneficial results.

Josh told me he was having additional symptoms that were distressing to him. His primary pain problems up to this time had been in his back, but now he was getting frequent severe headaches. He also had an almost continuous sensation of snapping and popping in the brain, and on several occasions had awakened in the morning feeling totally numb from the neck down, a feeling that lasted only a short time, perhaps half a minute. The first couple of times he thought he had dreamed it, but now he was sure it had really happened. With his usual understatement Josh said, "It's a bit scary."

His vision was causing him more trouble. His left eye, which was supposed to have been unaffected by the surgery, was becoming more and more difficult for him to focus. The vision in his right eye was far keener, he felt, than his left, although he had no peripheral vision in the right eye. He wondered whether it would be worth seeing an optometrist; perhaps glasses could help alleviate the vision distortion he was suffering. This was something positive we could do and I instantly agreed that we should pursue it.

The next week we went to an optometrist. The doctor found a measurable (though not great) difference in the vision of the two eyes and fitted him with glasses. After that, Josh wore them for reading or whenever he had to focus his eyes more acutely. The glasses didn't solve his problem entirely but they did help somewhat.

We were also busy during this time getting another new wig fitted for Josh. Now that he had some extra money from the sale of his car, he had decided to get a custom-made wig, hoping that it would be more comfortable and better-looking. After several fittings, the wig was finally ready. Although it was something of an improvement, it still did not look quite natural. But it was a more comfortable fit, partly because it was lightweight, so it became the one he wore most frequently. His hair had grown in quite thickly down the center, and now a softer type of hair, almost like baby fuzz, was growing in on the sides so that he did not look so bald. The distortion caused by the protruding flap was still quite noticeable, but much of it was covered by the hair on the top of his head, and people stared at him less frequently now. Even without added pressure his head hurt, so I encouraged him to forgo the wig whenever possible, and gradually, he began to go out without it. I always felt that even though his own hair did not look exactly right, he was much more himself when he didn't wear the wig.

The classes at Fernald were still the most important of Josh's outside activities. Moreover, he now had another interest there in addition to the tutoring he was receiving. Some months earlier, before Josh left for Europe, a new boy of about eleven or twelve named Don had been brought to the school. Fernald deals with emotional learning problems as well as physical ones, and this boy was hostile and belligerent—a real terror. Even his tutor seemed to have difficulty handling him, and the other teachers simply couldn't tolerate him at all. Josh determined to make friends with the boy. Alternately showing kindness and, when Don's behavior was too aggressive, indifference, he began to make inroads. Don showed less hostility toward Josh and gradually reached the point of actually demonstrating friendliness. He would show Josh the work he did in school and they always managed to chat for at least ten or fifteen minutes. Josh felt strongly that given adequate time, he could really help him to overcome some of his problems. He gave a lot of thought to Don and the way he was going to help him in the future.

Our days were taken up with doctors, Fernald, the wig, the glasses and the other errands we ran, but the evenings were very long indeed. Josh could no longer go to the movies because it was too uncomfortable for him to sit in the theater for any length of time. We could not take walks, but the weather wasn't pleasant anyway as Southern California was having heavy rainfall that autumn. It was as though the heavens themselves were weeping for Josh in his agony. During the evenings we now spent at home, we watched a little television, although Josh didn't care much for it, or we worked on Jumble puzzles, played Scrabble or just listened to music. Mostly, we would just talk and talk and talk. There was no subject that Josh and I did not discuss. I tried to keep the conversation interesting, tried to introduce new ideas to him, new concepts. One evening we had a long conversation about life after death and the numerous religious and mystical concepts concerning the immortality of the soul. Finally, after reviewing many different ideas on this matter, Josh decided that although none of them was believable, given a choice he'd opt for transmigration. Then, in unison, we both said, "And come back as Simon's son!" We had a stomach-knotting laugh over that. We'd show Sime—he couldn't just avoid Josh and get away free and clear!

When Josh was in a semi-reclining position in his chair, wearing his glasses and holding the Jumble book in his hand, he looked so nice, almost like a college boy again. Once in a while he would smile wanly at me and say, "Oh, Mash, Mash, look what you've done to me." I would look back at him and say, "Oh Josh, Josh, you've really blown it! How could you do this to your mother?" and we would laugh. He liked the repetition and we developed several repartees that we'd enjoy in almost ritual manner.

Josh was increasingly concerned about our financial situation. Since their return from Europe, Leib had been putting in extra long hours at work, but the results were quite meager. At this time, Josh began to spend perhaps half an hour or forty-five minutes each evening sketching an amusing cartoon representing Leib in different activities or postures, and he would write on it, "I am the Greatest" or "The Best Real Estate Man in the World." After Leib went to bed he would put these funny little creations either on the breakfast counter or in the bathroom for Leib to see in the morning. He was dedicated to encouraging his father and keeping his spirits up.

We returned for the other two acupuncture treatments on December 8 and 15. They provided no relief at all; if anything, Josh's back was hurting him more than before. The doctor admitted that there would be no use in pursuing this further; since the three treatments had produced no benefit, it was clear that the treatment would not be successful. Of course, it's possible that if we had had access to an expert Chinese practitioner, the results might have been better; but no such alternative was available to us. There was tremendous resistance on the part of the organized medical profession toward acupuncture. We availed ourselves of what UCLA had to offer, it did not work, and we accepted the fact that there was no help for Josh from this quarter.

*Ah, well, it's eleven-fifteen at night— almost midnight. Things are a little hard for me to remember; what — I want to say, or why I want to say them.*

*Questions like these are raised in my own mind. And, well, I'll try and think the best.*

*I'm having a little problem with my talking. Well, let me say a couple of things, get them out of my system, make me feel a little better. My back is—I don't like to use words like, "Oh, my back is killing me." Uh-uh, that's not the case—but something is wrong. I mean, I'm in severe pain.*

*I'm a little over twenty-one years old. That would have seemed to me an almost unimaginable amount of time. It's only been a little over one year since I've had some very interesting things happen to me, which I'll talk about at this particular moment. Ooooooh just trying to relax . . . Well, I don't know what I'm going to talk about first, but it helps, it really is physically helpful for me to say what I want to say. I can talk about whatever I want to talk about, because when they hear something like this in the future, it will perhaps be something strange, shocking, or something nice. It could be it's nice to hear; it could be good. I doubt that it could be bad.*

*Anyway, here I am again, Joshua Friedman, and I'm lying on my back. My back is— I'm very sore, very sore this evening. It's been very painful for some reason, I'd say this last week. I'll tell you what I'm talking about.*

*To get rid of that pain we just didn't know what to do— and it's getting so bad that I just can't do anything. I can't, uh, I can't, you know, move. I can't walk. It's hardly enjoyable, you know. What kind of enjoyment is this? Things are bad enough with my head, and I haven't been feeling well, but that kind of pain . . . it's out of hand. I just couldn't take it.*

*I went to see some gosh darned hick—he really was a hick, I think his name was Clyde; I don't know what his name was. A real turd. That was for my back. I don't know the correct term but when I explain it, you'll understand* it. It's like when they snap your back. I don't know, it begins with "ch-" [the initial sound in "chiropractor"]. Anyway they snap the parts in your back to straighten them out. It didn't work. There was another man, another fellow, who supposedly is really good. A lady at our apartment, one of our friends, suggested him because her husband had such a back pain and this other back snapper apparently helped. Anyway, we went to see another one [an osteopath] and that was no good. Let's see, that didn't do any good and the pains were just getting worse and worse in my back.

I better stop for a second because I'm having a little problem remembering. I'll start it right back up in a split second. Almost the same moment I turned this gizmo off, this set, this recorder, it just came back to me. It was called chemotherapy . . . No, no, no, it's the Chinese way to get rid of pain [acupuncture]. It's the yin and the yang, the yin and the yang. There are something like several hundred different parts in the body and by touching them with different pins the pain is sent over to another part; that's really not saying very much and I will try to fill you in. There are different parts of the body, like I told you. There are seven hundred to one thousand special points. It's an ancient art of getting rid of pain and apparently it's been working; but they don't know how, as for explaining it. It's very, very ancient and it really works. They've been using it from way back when. What they do is, they just stick pins in . . . they just stick those pins around your body. I went three times. We had this Jewish guy to work on me. He was the only one at UCLA who does this. His regular job, he was a doctor that puts you to sleep. I don't know the correct term [anesthesiologist]. I went three times and that thing didn't work. It's a combination of separate pins that they stick in to depths from very slight up to four inches deep. It didn't really hurt, it didn't hurt that much. It just was like beep! beep! but it wasn't really *bad. Unfortunately, it didn't do any good and it maybe seemed to make it a little worse for me. My system was just getting sorer and sorer so, uh, we just don't know what to say or do.*


There had to be some relief for Josh somewhere. Before we said good-bye to Dr. Levitz, I asked him if he knew of someone at UCLA who was working with hypnotherapy. Certainly, that was an approach that would not in any way interfere with any of the medical procedures, and it might be helpful to Josh. Happily, Dr. Levitz responded much more enthusiastically to this new idea of mine than Dr. Stark had to the acupuncture. He told me that he would get in touch with his friends at the Neuropsychiatric Institute and arrange for me to be contacted by someone there. However, it was now close to Christmas vacation and we would have to wait until after the first of the year.

The Fernald School closed for the Christmas vacation. With the coming of the middle of December we were faced with a couple of weeks of very limited activities. No school, no treatments. It was a very low point for us. Josh's pain had increased in intensity. The acupuncture hadn't helped and the results of the medicines were disappointing; all we could do was increase the amount of the narcotics he was taking. His associations at school, both with his tutor and with Don, were abruptly halted. The weather was wet, cold and miserable. Our autumn ended on a sad and depressing note.

# Winter 1973

Death is better than a life of pain, and
eternal rest than constant sickness.

Apocrypha, Ben Sira 30:17

*We're trying, we're working our hardest
— my parents and my brother and I are trying to make this
life a life that is a livable life, that's the right life, and we've
never really admitted to one another because we've kind
of kidded ourselves, but we knew—I think we knew.*

*This last has been a horrible thing, a horrible, horrible
thing. After what happened, we couldn't seem to — everybody was wonderful to me, they really were. They tried —
they were so concerned. Certain people . . . you are just
going to die at a certain age.*

Existence had become an almost unre-
lieved horror. Josh's pains were so severe that he was virtually incapable of movement without undergoing real
physical agony. The pain he suffered in his back, and now
in his head as well, was so intense that his sleeping was
disturbed and he would wake up frequently in order to
take additional medication. We went back to Dr. Goldman to try to get him some relief from the pain—something, anything. It no longer mattered how much medication he took as long as the pain was eased. Dr. Goldman
prescribed Thorazine and Demarol.

Josh rarely left the house; there was really nothing to
leave for. The Fernald School was closed for vacation, the
acupuncture treatments were over, and we were just waiting to hear from UCLA about hypnotherapy treatment.
Within two days after Josh started the new medications,
he was having periodic fits of melancholy and nausea. We

had to increase radically his intake of Valium to counteract the negative effect of these new drugs. I was thoroughly disheartened by what Dr. Goldman had done for Josh. There was no reduction of pain, but now Josh had the added problems of depression and frequent nausea.

I called Dr. Stark at the end of the week and described the new medications Josh was taking. Although he carefully controlled his response, I got the distinct impression that he was annoyed and angered that these medications had been given to Josh—particularly the Thorazine, which is not a pain depressant but is used for cases of mental unbalance. Dr. Stark gave me two prescriptions—one of them for codeine in larger quantities than Josh had previously received. Until now he had been taking three half-grain codeine pills every three to four hours. We now had a prescription for one-grain pills, and Josh started with two pills every three to four hours as he needed them; gradually, he was taking as many as three to four grains every four hours. At first, I resisted his taking the increased dosage but since anything less than three grains had no effect, and frequently even that did not provide adequate relief, I acquiesced. Josh was determined not to become totally immobilized by his pain.

*Medicines, man, do I take medicine! You can't believe how many medicines I take. If I didn't take any medicine, I wouldn't be anything, I'd be a nut. I'd be a piece of nothing. I'll stop right here, I don't want to say anything else, but . . . I take a lot of medicines.*

*Medicines concerning my head, different things to keep me alive and different things trying to cut down the pain. A lot, oh my Gosh! I don't know how many. I think we counted them up. We didn't count every one perfectly, obviously, but let's see, the last ten months, and I'm not* *talking like a fool, I mean, I'm not just saying things right off the top of the— See, right now I'm having problems, trying to understand things . . . I UNDERSTAND things but I'm having a hard time SAYING them when there should be no problem saying them. I try to relax and say them . . . I reckon in the last ten months, we have used up over one hundred thousand\* pills. Can you imagine? I've had to take so many pills just to keep me going during the day it's incredible. I need them, I need them for life. If I don't have them, especially the very, very important ones, I—Man! (snap) Bonk! I'd be right out of it! Take a nice little sleep there, ha! But, oh, wowee, that many pills! I mean you try to add it up, it's not exact, it might be off by fifteen or twenty, and I'm not kidding, but oh my gosh, it's been an awful lot.*

*We had a kind of a, a very sad thing happen just . . . um, I'm losing my bearings. Today is, let's call it Saturday, even though it's actually Sunday. It's midnight Saturday. Not last night, but the night before, uh, you know, I always keep in touch, calling people. It's been a very joyful thing to do . . . joyful? . . . enjoyable thing to do. I like to keep in touch with my relatives. I love people, elderly ones so much more. Not elderly, that's not a nice word. Older, older, that's it, yeah. We see them or call them.*

*These people, they used to live on Woodley Avenue. We lived there for about seven years, up until about a year ago, and we owned our big home there. We owned two other homes and we rented them. We had them stay there — my English isn't so good and I'm getting tired — an olderly couple. There was Jack and Betty. Kind of cute names, but they were really the nicest people. They loved each other, they were such an enamored love. They're both, I believe, sixty-two, sixty-three, something on that order; anyway, the*

---

\* Somewhat in excess of 10,000 would be more accurate.

*poor guy died. I called her two days ago — hadn't called her for a couple of weeks, and I called to say "hi." She told me that he was in the hospital . . . but things were OK now, I mean, he's going to get better. His weight had gone down, I don't know exactly, it's not that important, but the main thing is—the next day he died. Oh, it was so sad because I had just talked to her for quite a while, keeping her spirits up and everything like that. Everybody felt he would be better, and the next day he was gone, poor guy. The poor woman. You know, she's a nice lady.*

Josh developed an almost compulsive desire to purchase gifts for various members of the family, and for friends as well. Actually, between the middle of December and the start of the new year, about the only activities we had outside the house were shopping trips that Josh insisted we make, regardless of how uncomfortable he might be moving about. He bought holiday gifts for Simon and for me. He spent endless hours carefully comparing values and qualities of watches, and finally he purchased a very expensive wristwatch for Leib; it cost well over $100 and was by far the finest watch Leib had ever owned. He gave it to him with a sweet little speech explaining that it was a watch for a winner, not a loser; therefore, it would serve as a constant daily reminder to Leib that he was in fact "the greatest" and it would be a good talisman to help him in business. For Don, the little boy at school, Josh purchased a transistor radio as he knew that the boy's birthday was sometime during this holiday period. He went to great lengths to find what he felt was absolutely appropriate wrapping paper for a boy of that age, and he drew a simple and amusing card with just "Happy Brithday, Don" written on it so the boy would not have difficulty reading the message. The last time we had been to visit Dr. Marie, she had told Josh that she was planning to retire from practice in another month and that she and her husband and their family were moving to Greece. Josh bought a book on Greek art and also wrapped that himself to bring to her on our next visit. When we went on these shopping excursions, we tried to time them so that we would leave the house half an hour to forty-five minutes after he had taken his pain pills. He would then have an hour or two that, while not totally free of pain, was less intensely uncomfortable than other times. Frequently, as we walked, he was so overcome with shooting pains that he would have to lean on me. We must have made a strange-looking pair: a tall, skinny, peculiarly awkward young man stooped over and leaning on a short, middle-aged woman. Josh would set goals for himself, mountains to conquer. "Mom, I don't care what it costs me in pain. I've decided to walk at least one whole block. You don't mind my leaning on you, do you?" For me, it was indescribable pain of a different sort—to watch him suffer so, trying so hard not to give in to the pain.

One of the real joys in which he could still thoroughly immerse himself was listening to music. He decided to get a better FM radio than the one he already had, which was adequate for pop songs but did not have the precision or tone quality to do justice to classical music. He purchased a fairly good Sony radio and it was at this time that I bought the cassette recorder which he was later to use in making his tapes.

It was a period that we spent in a strange sort of isolation, particularly for that time of the year. Simon did not come home for Christmas vacation. We received very few social invitations for the holidays and planned no dinners or parties since Josh was so uncomfortable most of the time that I wasn't sure in advance when he could enjoy company.

The one social function we decided Josh would enjoy

235

was a brunch my friend Charlotte was giving on Christmas Day. Her four boys and my two were quite close in age. Charlotte and I have been friends since we were teenagers, and although we have never lived close to one another, over the years the children had seen each other fairly often, particularly on holidays or other special occasions. The boys, though not good personal friends, were rather like extended family—distant cousins perhaps. I thought Josh might like seeing the four boys and the new baby of the oldest and that he could feel completely relaxed in Charlotte's home. Charlotte had visited us frequently throughout the course of his illness and Josh was at ease in her company.

As it turned out, Josh felt surprisingly good that day, but the boys were simply unable, as I had noticed with so many other young people throughout the development of Josh's illness, to make natural contact with him. The short conversations were awkward and stilted. Oh, they were polite. They spoke a few meaningless sentences with him, but basically they avoided him. I had seen this so many times before; it was as though the ill person had become in some way ritually impure and was almost taboo. Whether it is out of embarrassment or fear or guilt, I do not know. There is, however, a pervasive pattern of treating terminally ill people almost as though they don't exist. They become, in effect, nonpersons. Perhaps this avoidance makes the healthy feel less personally threatened by death. Certainly to the person who is ill, such behavior appears painfully obvious and clumsy. He begins to feel that perhaps it would be better not even to attempt to communicate with others, but rather to withdraw and limit one's conversation and exchange of ideas to his immediate family and the doctors.

Josh tried. He spoke to each of them individually for a moment or two, but the conversations were so labored and the responses so halting that finally he just gave up trying. We stayed a polite amount of time and then went home.

The next day Josh received a visit from his best friend, Jeff, who came in the afternoon and stayed about an hour and a half. He hadn't been to see Josh in over five months. Josh was not well enough to go out, so they stayed in his room. He gave Jeff his old FM radio, which he no longer needed, and at about five o'clock Jeff left with a smiling good-bye and a promise to visit Josh again very soon. I invited him to stay for dinner, but he had other plans. It was the last time Josh saw him. Josh had missed him terribly, but now, having seen him again, he did not seem disappointed when Jeff left. Josh had grown apart in so many ways from the normal existence Jeff still led that there was no longer any real area of mutual interest.

The last few days of the year were endless twenty-four-hour cycles of pain, isolation and loneliness. Shortly before the New Year I called Dr. Levitz, the acupuncturist, and asked if he had been able to find out anything about a hypnotherapist for Josh. He assured me that he had made inquiries but had not yet been able to set up anything specific. However, he promised to get back to us early in January.

New Year's Eve, we three—Leib, Josh and I—spent at home, much like any other evening. Even Josh's recliner was uncomfortable for him, so at about nine in the evening he went to lie down on his bed, listen to music, and work some of his Jumble puzzles. I offered to sit with him in his room and keep him company, but he didn't want that. Leib and I were reading in the living room. I kept wondering how it was possible that nobody, nobody at all, had called Josh to wish him a Happy New Year. None of his friends called, and of the relatives in the area only my parents had called, earlier in the day. I remember sitting with the book open in front of me, not really reading, but feeling so angry, so unbearably bitter that even before his death it seemed as though my son was already forgotten— forgotten by those who claimed to love him, to be concerned. From time to time, I looked in on Josh, offered him something to drink or a piece of fruit. I sensed that he was probably experiencing very similar thoughts to mine. He really didn't want me there to watch him for fear that he might demonstrate bitterness or what he had so earnestly avoided for ten months now, any show of self-pity.

At about five minutes past midnight the phone rang. It was our wonderful friends from Belgium, Annette and Roger, calling to wish us all, and particularly Josh, a Happy New Year. I couldn't speak with them, nor did I even want to. It was too costly and too wonderful to waste on me. After Leib spoke for a few moments, we carried the phone into Josh's room and Josh spoke with them for perhaps five minutes. There could have been no sweeter gesture; nothing else at that particular moment could have reversed Josh's mood as that telephone call did. When the call was over, Josh got up from bed and came into the living room and we all had a glass of wine together, toasting each other a Happy New Year—as happy as we could make it.

Leib went to bed, and Josh and I sat up and talked. He was in a good frame of mind and told me that he had made a New Year's resolution. It was quite simple. He was going to do as much as he could with every day of his life that was left. Having told me that, quite happily, he went to bed.

With the start of the new year, and in line with Josh's resolution, we resumed some of the activities that had come to a halt. Things were no longer the same, however. Josh's condition was declining in many ways, and he was now constantly in pain. Even with the larger doses of codeine, there were only a few short stretches of time during

238

the course of any day that he found tolerable. His actions were limited to sitting upright or walking the short distance downstairs to the car, or from the car to the classroom at Fernald or in and out of a doctor's office. Anything beyond that was simply too painful for him to bear. We saw Dr. Marie and Josh gave her the book he had bought for her. We kept in close touch with Dr. Goldman, for no other purpose—since I no longer trusted his judgment—than to get constant renewals of the codeine prescription. We had some family visitors at the apartments, and Josh tried hard on those occasions to sit up and really visit with them but without a great deal of success. His appetite had left him and he was losing weight quite noticeably. I did whatever I could to stimulate his appetite, to encourage him to eat, but to little avail.

He now frequently missed classes at Fernald. So many days he just didn't have the energy to rise above the pain and get to school. On the days he did attend, he was seldom able to stay much longer than an hour. As always, as he had done since he first started school, he would tell me how the lessons went and what they had done. I could see from what Josh told me that Barbara was responding to his obvious decline by imposing very few demands on him. Actually they spent most of the time playing Scrabble or other word games or just talking. They were no longer working with the machines or trying to increase the speed of his reading.

Early in the month, Dr. Levitz called me from UCLA and gave me the name of a man to call about hypnotherapy, a Mr. Green. He was someone working on experimental programs at the Neuropsychiatric Institute, a lay hypnotist, not a medical man, but apparently he had repeatedly demonstrated a really extraordinary ability to assist people, particularly the physically ill, with hypnosis. His efforts had proved beneficial not only in controlling pain, but in some cases had improved patients' recuperative abilities. I called Mr. Green, gave him an outline of Josh's case and made an appointment.

I prepared Josh by telling him, truthfully, that I felt hypnotherapy was a technique that had unmeasured and untapped potential for pain control and even for cure. I genuinely believe that as we learn more about somatic self-control, not only through auto-hypnosis, but through various other latent mental capacities, man will exert greater power over his own body. A tentative step in this direction, I told him, had been made in some studies being done with alpha waves—no mystical nonsense, strictly scientific demonstrations. As a result of my preparation, Josh approached hypnotherapy with very positive thoughts.

During our initial visit, Mr. Green spent a considerable amount of time detailing his personal background and training in hypnotherapy. I can't quite decide whether this was done from a sense of pride in his accomplishments or to justify and sanction his work—perhaps a bit of both.

He was, as I have said, not a doctor, and had no medical training. His interest in hypnosis dated back some thirty years, when he was a vaudeville musician and had become intrigued by hypnotist acts he watched. He felt this was something he could do, so he studied hypnosis and became quite successful as a performer. Five or six years later, he became gravely ill. Applying to himself the techniques he had previously used only for entertainment, he became extraordinarily adept at auto-hypnosis and made an incredible recovery from his illness. After that experience he became interested in hypnosis as a scientific discipline, read widely in the literature, and worked many years to maximize his own control. Eventually he was able not only to exclude pain totally from his consciousness but to control his rate of respiration, heartbeat and blood pressure. He had completely stopped thinking of hypnosis in terms of entertainment and had become a professional practicing hypnotherapist.

Mr. Green explained to Josh that the treatment would involve nothing more than lying down, relaxing and permitting the therapist to make contact with his subconscious through hypnosis. If Josh could cooperate and not resist him, then he could conceivably bring him a good deal of relief. Josh was more than willing to try. He would have done anything within reason to find some way of controlling the interminable pain he suffered.

Actually, however, Josh proved to be a poor subject. I think there were several reasons for this. First of all, Mr. Green was much more tentative in his approach to hypnotizing Josh than he normally was with other patients. It was his first time working with a brain-damaged person and he told me he was just a bit wary of leaning too hard, of being too forceful, as he might do some harm from lack of knowledge in this particular case. Secondly, Josh was by nature not given to letting go of his control. This was the key to his entire magnificent performance throughout his illness—this determination of his to maintain control. But it worked against him in his sessions with the hypnotist. Also, by this time I think it may have been too late for hypnotherapy to work. Josh's comprehension had been much reduced in the preceding month or two, and he found it difficult to remember all the preparatory material Mr. Green repeated to him each time before actually trying to get Josh into a state of hypnosis. Therefore, much of the time that should have been spent in working with Josh in deeper hypnotic states was used to go over the preliminary explanations. After several sessions Mr. Green saw this as a primary problem in getting through to Josh. Finally, he made some tapes for us in the hope that Josh, by listening to them frequently at home, might better grasp the basic orientation and therefore derive greater benefit from the actual sessions.

*I've been going for some hypnosis. Ah! Ah! you're wondering about that wild kid, that wild child. Joshy, Joshy what are you doing—who are you, who are you? . . . It's nothing like that, this is all seriousness. Well, I'll talk about it, anyway. I believe it was Monday, Wednesday and Friday—anyway, three times now I've been going to a hypnotic or hypnotist, if that's the correct word. Anyway, the reason is that I've been having pain. As a matter of fact, I have a little problem in my own brain, with some mixing up, and I sometimes forget things very quickly. But I think we've heard this thing over and over and sometime it will make sense. I have a little problem myself.*

*The latest thing we've been trying is this, uh, using a hypnotist and hypnotism. It's been tested, I mean, it's been well known in the 1900's. I've been having this, having this hypnotism a couple of times now. We're at the end of January now, 1973, and I think we might be able to get rid of some of that pain. The pain will still be there, but mentally I won't have it there anymore. I'll be able to send it away. There might be something wrong. I might have a back tumor growing in me now. We've gone many, many times to these doctors for this and for that; we can't find anything bad or any growth on my back but it's been very, very bad. They don't know everything. I will take anything at the moment, you know, I've just got to get rid of this pain. So we'll try this and hope that it works. Anyway, I've talked a little bit about the doctors and stuff and I've kept you up on what's going on. I really hope that this will work.*

*Let's see the other things that I have been doing. Well, you know, the pain is, I have been talking a lot about the back, but with the head, well, we've got to talk a little about that. Unfortunately we can't stop it growing. We don't know what day it's going to be that . . . That's it but, that's pretty much what we've been told. I try and do things when I can. I am pretty much stuck with my mother. Once in a while I go with my father and there really isn't a heck of a lot to do. It isn't the most exciting life to lead, but, thank goodness, I have such a fantastically intelligent genius of a mother; it's great to have a mother with an IQ who can keep up with things that are learned and found out and things like that. I don't know about my father exactly; he is a very, very bright man. He's done well and things like that, you know. But she's a reader; she reads so much. She reads two full books every evening. She was, at one time, just several years ago, finally going to get her PhD. I don't know what she would have wanted to do afterwards, write a fantastic this or that—I don't know what. Some super thesis. Anyway, she decided not to finish that. She is just pretty much concerned with me now. I don't . . . I can't do that much you know. When things are at their best I can't wait to go someplace. She drives; once in a while I drive. It depends on what we can do. But there isn't really that much to do, or that much that's exciting to do, and we really can't go very far because I've got such bad back pains. I can't do anything that's for the physically strong or that's ridiculously enjoyable, but we do what we can. We go to see movies. You know, I've always loved to see movies. I've wanted to make films. I mean, I've made a couple of little films and I got a nice camera, but thinking of becoming a filmmaker, no, no, no, that's not what's needed. I'd like to go and do filming. I've done it and it's fun, but I can hardly go anywhere. Before I go, you know I can't go far, that's what I'm trying to say, I can't go far . . .*

*Anyway, there's not much that I do. I wasn't able to go see any movies, since I, oh gosh, since I came back from*

*Europe, and that was, oh, three or four months ago. You
know, I just can't go anywhere. I like to see movies, but
ooooh those aching pains. So I, uh, what we do is try to do
other things. I've started to play some Scrabble. I know
that I am . . . I know that the correct word is not that I am
a supergenius but I'm definitely of genius caliber like, I believe, my mother and her sister. My mother is about forty-
seven now and her sister Ruth is about fifty, she is fifty and
my mother is forty-seven and they are both extremely intelligent women. This is not one of those cases when you're
proud and brag about it when there is no justification. In
this case it is really the truth. They are so bright, unbelievably bright; they know anything. You just ask them anything
and they just yappety, yappety—they can tell you just anything you want to know. They've always been great readers,
from the very beginning. As children they were— Instead
of graduating high school at the normal age of eighteen,
they were out at fourteen or fifteen — those kinds of
things. They . . . are just fantastic people. So, to have a
mother like this, to be able to see her all the time, we talk
about, about this and that. I mean I'm always learning
things. Since she was married to Leib, you mix those genius
brains together and you wind up with a Joshua and a Simon
Friedman. You know, there is a lot of brains! It's in my
system, I know, I know so much, and they've done it to me.*

We went three times a week for the rest of January and
into the beginning of February. Josh did not really benefit
in the sense of actually achieving any measurable ability to
induce self-hypnosis. However, he did feel he was making
progress and wanted to continue the sessions. A couple of
times during a session, Josh would experience very brief
periods of remission from pain; it gave us some hope,
although there was no lasting resolution to his suffering.

Aside from the continuing pain and weight loss, Josh seemed to be suffering a more general sort of debility. He was tired all the time and his vision gave him increasing difficulty. He became so sensitive to light that it was necessary for him to wear sunglasses. I noticed that his coordination was deteriorating from its best postsurgical level, and he frequently bumped into objects, even walls, when walking.

Almost more disturbing than the physical manifestations were subtle behavioral changes. Early in February he started to spend some time making little repairs around the apartment. He rewired the hookup for the television so that some of the fuzziness was eliminated. He repaired a lamp that one of the cats had knocked over and which had been unstable. As he did many things like this around the apartment, I began to sense an extraordinary similarity to the kind of feeling one has during the last month of pregnancy before entering the hospital; it is as though certain things must be accomplished while there is still time. Josh didn't verbalize this, but it was clear from his pattern of behavior that he was trying to get things finished.

Early in February he again brought up the subject of disposal of his body by cremation. I assured him that I not only remembered my promise but had even made inquiries. Cremation is not normally encouraged, or even accepted, among Jews, so I looked for an alternative to the customary Jewish mortuary. I had heard of an organization called Telophase which arranged for cremation and I called to request a brochure about their service. In about a week, the brochure and an application form arrived in the mail. We examined the material together, and I explained that his signature would be required to affirm that he wished this procedure to be followed upon his death. Very determinedly he signed the application, also indicating that he wished his ashes to be scattered at sea. With an obvious air of something "well done" he mailed back the form.

After our tenth visit to the hypnotherapist, Josh thought he had finally broken through the principal barriers restraining him from truly benefiting from the treatment. He felt that he finally grasped the basic nature of what was being attempted. As he saw it, anything he set his mind to do, if he wanted it badly enough and believed in it thoroughly enough, he would be able to do. The next day, February 8, with this new determination, this new concept of his own untapped ability to do something beyond what would normally appear possible, he decided that he wanted to take a long drive—with himself at the wheel! He was certain he was capable of doing this and that it would be the best treatment for him. He was so happy, so positive, so forceful in this determination that I agreed enthusiastically.

We decided to drive to Sun City to visit his grandparents and aunt. We left the house very early for us—dressed, breakfasted and in the car by ten-thirty. Josh made the two-hour drive without a murmur, without any expression of physical discomfort. He was so intent in the physical act of driving that for those two hours he literally felt no pain. This was the first time Josh had driven for over a month; because of the pain, he had not even asked to drive. I saw at once that he now had greater depth-perception and distance-distortion problems, but he drove very carefully and there was not much traffic at that time of day. When we arrived at my parents' home, it was clear that the ride had given him a tremendous sense of achievement and gratification.

He was tired but very happy. I insisted that he lie down and take a little rest. This he did with no argument at all and actually fell asleep for an hour. After that we all went out to eat and then I drove us home. Josh was happier and more lively that day than he had been for weeks. He felt so proud that he was able to overcome his pain and demonstrate such capability.


*I, myself, just am lying down. The reason I'm laying down is to make myself feel better, that's absolutely nothing, right? That's right. I have got some pain that I just don't know anything about, don't know why I've got that pain, but dammit, it really is hurting. Pain can be very, very, very destroying. Having pain all the time, continually, continuing to hurt makes things bad. This pain can make your whole system worth nothing. Intense pain can make you feel so unhappy. It's hard to get the correct word across. I'm using every bit I can to get that damn pain out of my system, so I don't feel it; then I can have a nice, lovely discussion concerning something. Now I'm hoping we can, when I say we, I'm speaking of myself, I'm in my room, I've turned off the light and I'm lying back. It's time to go to bed, it's, I reckon, about twelve-thirty. I want to get rid of this pain. We have tried everything to get rid of this pain but to no avail.*

*The last few weeks I have been going for hypnotism. I believe I've mentioned it before and I had taped it. I'm very sure I have. We think it has proven to help to a certain degree, maybe a very minor, miniscule, whatever the word is, amount, I think it is helping to some degree and it's very important that I keep these recordings because in the future, looking back, I'll know whether I have made some progress concerning this pain or not. I'm just breathing, just breathing, trying to relax, to get that pain out of here. This pain is enough to just ruin your system. It's enough to . . . it's so horrible, this pain. I'm just talking now, because in all honesty, I just keep myself talking to get rid of that pain. If I turn this device off, this recorder, oh my*

*gosh, I don't want to even think about it. I just want to
talk about anything to keep that pain out of here. This
pain is enough to just drive you — oh . . . I'm quite certain
that if I keep talking to myself, which makes a recording,
later on I'll be able to get myself interested in my own
thoughts and oh, discuss something. I'm positive it won't
be interesting, but it makes me feel better. I feel like a
knife — sharp in my system. I mean, cut it out!!! My back,
whooooooo, go! go! go! Right now, I'm not even remembering but I'm going to work at it, and I'll get my memory
back.*

That Sunday, February 11, Simon came home for the
day. His nineteenth birthday was the following day and
Josh and I had bought him presents. It had been some
time since his last visit, and I think I *really* saw for the first
time how terribly Josh had declined in observing Simon
with him. First of all, Simon's face plainly showed disbe-
lief at the degree of deterioration. Secondly, and more painfully, I had been so alone with Josh, so isolated, that I had
almost no frame of reference by which to gauge his physical and mental condition. When I saw him with my
healthy son, I realized how very much worse Josh was. It
was almost a relief when Simon left. It had been too painful to see the two of them together. They had been, when
Josh was well, so much alike. Now Josh, except for his
height, was so diminished in every way. He was very thin
and weak, and was having so much renewed difficulty with
his speaking—it had all sort of slipped up on us without
our being aware of how drastic the changes were.

The next day, Josh did not feel well enough to go to
Mr. Green for his hypnotherapy session. On Tuesday, I
called the Fernald School to tell them that Josh didn't feel
up to going for a lesson. Then, on Wednesday, Josh suf-

fered a partial paralysis while shaving in the morning. Quite suddenly, and without pain, the right side of his body became numb. He could not control the movements of his right arm. He could walk but his right leg dragged. His speech was partially slurred, as though he had suffered a stroke. I called Dr. Stark and spoke with his nurse, describing the partial paralysis and the difficulty he had been having with his vision. I distinctly remember her saying, "Oh, poor Josh." It was the only time during the year that I heard this woman in any way indicate a personal reaction to anything I told her. At that moment I knew this was the end. That "Oh, poor Josh" had slipped out, so spontaneously. I knew she was instinctively reacting to what she must have seen with many other patients over the years. We set up an appointment to see the doctor the next day.

Surprisingly, the paralysis seemed totally gone the next morning. Josh's speech was clear, he was able to use his right arm and, although his right hand itself had lost its grasping strength, it was responsive in every other way. There was nothing more Dr. Stark could do for him other than check him over, hear his description of the new symptoms, and generally just reassure Josh that he was there and available to be of what help he could. There were no promises made. Had there been, they would have been obvious falsehoods. I took this occasion, seeing the doctor face-to-face rather than speaking by telephone to tell him again that the pain Josh was suffering was growing more intolerable with each passing day. I told him how much codeine we were now giving Josh and suggested that he would soon need a more powerful narcotic. Now that Josh had suffered a partial (although temporary) paralysis, and with the increasing vision distortion, it wasn't necessary for the doctor to tell us that there wasn't a great deal of time left.

Dr. Stark said, "There is only one other thing we can do for Josh. When the pain reaches the point that is absolutely and unquestionably intolerable, we can hospitalize him and give him morphine injections to ease the pain." He paused, waiting for a response from me.

"What will that really mean, doctor?"

"Mrs. Friedman," he said, "it's our experience that in order to administer adequate morphine to successfully combat the extreme pain Josh will be suffering we will probably have to reach dosages that ultimately will inhibit his other bodily functions."

"In other words, you're telling me he'll get so much morphine that it will stop his respiration and heart function? It will be the end?"

"Yes, that's right," he said.

The rationale for this procedure is, I suppose, that one is treating the patient for pain. The unspoken promise is that once the patient has reached the point where, not only is there no hope, but the pain is beyond bearing, he will be slowly killed under the guise of being helped to bear the pain. I asked the doctor, "How long does this usually take?"

He said, "Three to four days."

"But Josh won't suffer? He won't be in pain?" I pleaded.

"No, no pain."

Leib had come with us to the doctor for this appointment. He was as alarmed as I at the paralysis Josh suffered and I wanted him with us when we spoke to the doctor. After we left the office, the three of us drove to the beach to a cafe overlooking the ocean. Josh wanted to know what the doctor had said beyond what he had understood. I told him as carefully and as explicitly as I could. I explained that when his discomfort reached the point that he could not tolerate it, the doctor would help him. He could go to the hospital and they would give him morphine so that he would feel no further pain. That was a promise—it was also going to be the end. Josh accepted this very well and couldn't understand why the doctor hadn't told him directly. To Josh this was not a negative statement but a positive one. There was a way out.

Josh said, "I know I'm getting very close to the end now. But this is okay—this is an okay way to go." The paralysis had been a most disconcerting development, he was having so much difficulty with his vision and coordination, and the pain was constantly mounting. He didn't want us to feel badly because, as he said, "I've really had quite enough."

I told him, "Josh, that's your choice and you're entitled to make it. But let's just make a real effort to do everything you still can do. Don't precipitate the final decision."

*February 17, 1973*

*Well, it's another one of those lovely days. Seems like, seems like everything is a total fiasco. Things seem to never get any better, just worse. I'll talk about them a little bit.*

*Last Thursday, it was two days ago, we had to go to see Dr. Stark, the brain surgeon. We went at one o'clock and there was myself, and my mom and dad. We know, basically, that things are going pretty much to the end, but they get worse. We don't know what it's going to be like. Even though I know things are going to get worse and worse and worse, the way he says it is pretty disgusting. I don't want to sound like that, I don't mean to sound like that, I don't mean to sound like that — as a matter of fact, I won't change anything. I'm just gonna keep going. . . .*

*Just one of those perfectly happy days! When we saw Dr. Stark, you know each time I've seen him it's been . . . I haven't seen him for probably two weeks— two months. Before that, gosh, over the months I've seen him very often. When I was in Intensive Care for five weeks, God, I saw that guy so much during the day. Since everything was . . . felt kind of strange anyway . . . it was unbelievable* how much time I spent seeing this guy. Since he'd operated and tried to get rid of the tumor, afterwards, for the first four, or even five weeks, I just couldn't get rid of that guy's name. When I say I couldn't forget it, first I couldn't remember it. No matter how many times—no matter how, no matter how many times—numbers and numbers and numbers and numbers of times, I just couldn't remember it. Then, afterward, when I finally got it, there'd be no way to ever forget it, it was there.

Anyway, this last Thursday we went to the doctor. We hadn't been there in two weeks— two months, and we knew things were very bad and . . . you know something? He used to be a different kind of man in our minds; in my dad's mind, in my mind, but things haven't really changed a bit. When we found out what was going on, well it was pretty— He wasn't even talking to me . . . he didn't— He was a louse. He wasn't a real man who would tell ME . . . You know, he would tell my folks and then they . . . Of course he'd leave—and Mom and Dad would have to do it. My English isn't good — I don't even worry about that. I mean, that's nothing new, I've already mentioned that. He was—it just wasn't very, very nice of him to do that. He could have told me. But the only time he told me was when I was just about getting out of the office and then I wouldn't be able to see him. He just zooped out, and that's not very nice.

Anyway, we've been going to the hospital and we found out what's wrong and I mean it's just unfortunate. It's getting worse and worse and there's nothing you can do. But he's kind of a . . . what's that word? I'll call it a shit, OK? You know, he could have . . . still things haven't changed . . . At that time, especially, I told you Dad and I thought he was the greatest and Mom did, too. Wow, he's saving me my life. If I had a million dollars, I'd give it out, right away. Well, ha! ha! it didn't do any good, ha. Now Dad is

. . . . you can see he . . . my dad is pretty disgusted with him, like I am. He's a . . . he will never tell me anything—no, he always has to tell Mom and Dad and then he can just zip out. That's not very . . . that's not fine, not fine for him to act like that.

Anyway, um, this last Thursday was when we saw him and I wasn't too happy to see him because I used to think he was the greatest, but he really isn't. Obviously, we knew that people die, that's all there is to it. I know—I know he's not a perfect man, but he is good; not everybody lives. Obviously, I'm one of the ones that, apparently, can't or won't. But it isn't—he can't . . . He acts a certain way, for a time, for a couple of times, days and days until I'm out of Intensive Care and I'm out of the hospital, but then after that he just kind of forgets about it, goes to the other people. He doesn't keep up with what's going on. Other things are apparently more important in his mind. When I saw him Thursday, he — he's— We used to think of him as such a nice — he's a God, Mom and Dad and me thought; but now he's anything but. We knew from the very beginning he was always a salty-looking guy, never a smile on his face, but we accepted that. At least he was something, he was a unique man and the finest. But I don't know now. I have no love for this guy. It's just not lovely to hear now or think about it.

One more time, my English is not coming out too good. So we saw him and— What I wanted to talk about is, well, let's say, things are worse and worse. Now, these last few days, just about a week ago, things really haven't — I haven't been feeling too good. My head has been really, really, really been hurting me, which is nothing new, but it's been quite a few weeks that I haven't really gotten such bad headaches. They would go—you know they would come and then they'd go for quite a while. They'd come and go.

Anyway, we were talking about Dr. Stark and he's a little salty old man. Most people, either their face is straight or with a built-in smile even if they close their mouth, it's kind of a smile. His is extremely the opposite. He's just quite upside-down. If he was laughing, it would be just a straight line, and it wouldn't even look like a laugh. Anyway, we went to the doctor and things weren't good. Fine, that's nothing new, but apparently, things do get worse and sometimes . . . I can go so quick.

Last week, boy, things just really started coming bad. For several, several weeks, things were pretty damn good. I went— I did the driving and I did everything that I could. We didn't go to a helluva lot of places but we did the best we could and enjoyed the best we could. About a week ago, things got really bad. I'll talk about a few of these things. One of them . . . Let's start off with my head. My gosh, you know, these headaches are real bad, we don't know about this. I mean every hour I have to take asperins and codeine and they're just not doing it—they're real bad. So, that is one thing that is real bad. Second . . . secondly, my back—it's intensive. Thirdly, the . . . I'm losing my . . . the third of the things that I'll mention is — I'm kind of losing things . . . I can't control things. Put it this way, this is the third time now, or fourth time . . . At first I didn't really realize, is this real or not? The first time you ever feel anything you forget it. It goes away; you always forget about it. The second time, too. The third time, then you go, "Oh yeah, that's how I feel." Anyway, the second time, it felt like I was kind of losing my control, in the sense that —well, put it this way. If you had a seizure or something on that order, certain people, they just fall down, they just have no control. Well this is not what I've got. What I feel now, I feel numb. What I'm trying to say is my numbness is like . . . If you've ever had a shot for your tooth—can't remember the word, what's it called? [Novocaine.] Supposing you get a toothache, they give you something and you don't feel it at all and then they fix your teeth and then, in a couple of hours it gets good again. It's kind of like that, except my back. Both my hands and arms were kind of— numb. I wasn't out of control. It wasn't like not being able to understand what it was; I did. When it's almost all numb, it's hard to see what you're talking about. It's not as bad as not having any control and you can't move your hand at all. It's a little bad. Anyway, that was the second time, but the third time, which was last night, it's been kind of bad. My right side, I want to make this quite clear, it's getting numb. Late last evening, it got kind of, I just kind of lost control of . . .

I gotta say this. My eye—if I were to look at anything on the right side, I don't see anything. If it's anything slightly off middle all the way over to the right, because after the . . . when I had the major operation . . . I can't see on the right side. Most of the time, I can see anything on the left side, but on the right side, unless I turn my head around to see it, I wouldn't see it. Anyway, on that side, I can't see* . . . What am I talking about? Oh well . . . It feels like, certain things have to come and go . . .

The right hand now is kind of . . . I don't see it to begin with unless I turn my head, but regardless, if I do look at it, it's hard to have as much control as a normal hand. Now the left side, is working fine, it's just normal. But on the right side, like last night and all day today, it's like I don't have all a hundred per cent control, you know what I mean? I don't have any pain, I reckon, it comes and goes. But if there's no pain, I don't know where the heck I really am. Apparently, things are getting worse, that's what Dr. Stark talks about. It's getting worse. We— The first day I thought I felt a little something, but it was nothing. The

* He was having difficulty seeing in any direction at this point.

second time, both of my fingers were a little bit bowed. The third one, which is last night and today, Saturday— no—yeah—the left is fine, the one on the right, I— kind of it hurts—like I don't have a hundred per cent control there. Anyway Stark told me about it and he said it's gonna get worse and worse. I mean, I could lose control until I have nothing. I mean, I could be paralyzed and everything could be completely gone. Just lose everything and this pain is—the pain hasn't been too bad today.

Mom, you've listened to this and Dad, you've listened to this—you know what's going on. We don't know if the thing gets really, really, sourly painful and I just have no way to do it. I mean, they cannot put me to sleep but, apparently they do. I found out. They told me. They give you morphine and you have no pain; that's something, you have no pain. You don't even remember where you are and in three or four days it kills you, but you won't have any horrible pain, no pain at all.

Exactly a year ago, I went — I — after I was in Intensive Care, then when I finally got out of Intensive Care, I don't remember how long it was, a week or whatever, they put me in a regular room, you know, there was me and some other man. But after that, something just went right out because apparently, I didn't know this, the next thing I knew, I was back in Intensive Care. You see, that was when they had cut my— had to open everything up and work on it or something like that.

I was in— Even though I was in a regular room, I didn't know about this — it was either three and a half or four days, I didn't know it. Something went wrong, I didn't know. My pain was so bad; it didn't stop for over three days. I didn't want to make a sound, scream or anything, but I was just—they couldn't do it; they were giving me as much morphine but still the pain. It hasn't been doing anything. Can you imagine? That pain was so intense, so

gosh darn painful. They had to cut on me and everything.
I didn't know it. I was so screwed up, my system was so
goofed up, they had to give me that morphine to have— to
get rid of some of that pain—they didn't stop the pain. I
was in so bad pain; but it doesn't matter, don't you worry
about it, Mom or Dad, because that's way back then, a
year ago, and I didn't even know about it. Pain, big deal,
it doesn't matter. But, should this happen and we can't get
that pain out, they can at least give me something. If I'm
crippled, or if the pain is so bad I can't know where I am,
it'll be three or four days, but I won't have the pain, or at
least, hopefully, it won't be that bad.

Also today, I might mention that I want to be — what's
the . . . let's see if I can remember, I have a hard time —
cremated, yeah that's— I told my folks many, many
months ago that, should I die, I want to be cremated. That
means when I've died, and it's all over, I don't want any
pieces or parts or any of that stuff. After that day, cremate
me; that means it burns it all up, there's nothing left. Then
they just throw pieces of—just little pieces of ashes, just a
little bit up in the sky . . . It'll be quick, and be sooner that
we get it out of your system. You'll know of me and you'll
think highly of me and proudly; but you won't have the
bad removal — re — re — the things that you remember.
It burns everything clear. Its' very pleasant and besides, ha!
ha! you don't have to come over and visit me.

I just took all these medicines . . . came back up! I've
been laying down, standing up — different — I'm not feeling good now, I'm really losing control over my right— It's
going— Where is it? I'll look to the left. OK, now I have
control at least on the left. Hey, this is no joke! But at least
I'll take it like a goddamn man.

Yes, in my right labe— labe— My reading's [speaking]
going bad; sometimes when I read [speak], I can't even
control those . . . You can see my English is wrong, my

*English has been bad, it goes up . . . and bad and worse and worse. I don't feel good. I wonder if I can at least make it on the right. I'm gonna try. Yeah, where was I? Some control with my English. Oh boy! I'm not disgusting, I'm just unhappily—whoops, where is it? Ohhh——*

*Suddenly I just don't feel too well. I'll talk another time and mention the important things. The main thing is, besides the pain, the— the loss of control of one side or the other, or both, and the pain and all these goodies—there is nothing we can do about it.*

*But I knew, back when—I think it was about two years ago* [at the time of Abe's death and cremation] *I said to myself, "Who knows? It would be possible that I know that within a year, I'll die." I mean, I knew that, well, a year ago—no, two years ago, first, I'd remembered and I— Suppose I had heard that I was going to die and I only had a year. I was ready for it before this; before we even found out all this stuff. I really did say, "Suppose I heard that I was going to die, that I had a year"; I was really quite ready. Then after a year, exactly a year, then I did get the word. So it's been a year, and things have really been going pretty well straight down the class — down the class — well, I don't know the correct word. I'd better just stop for the moment, because I'm not feeling good. I just wanted to mention some of the things that I talked about. It was— well, on and off—it'll be later in the evening—it's a quarter to nine so I'll say good-bye . . .*

We agreed that, having nothing left to lose, we would again increase Josh's codeine intake. He started taking four to five grains every few hours, and for the next couple days he seemed able to move around more comfortably. The numbness on his right side and the inability to control precise movements with his right hand came and went several times during the course of each day.

Josh called Simon and asked him to come home; he wanted to see him. Simon came up the next Sunday and Josh had him read back to him all the mail he had received over the course of the past year. Josh checked to make sure there was no unanswered mail, and then they carefully bundled the letters and put them away in a desk drawer.

After Simon left that Sunday, Josh started calling all the relatives and family friends he had been in contact with during the year. He managed during the next two or three days to speak with each of them and then put a check beside the name in his address book.

As the week progressed, we found it impossible to leave the apartment. Josh's pain, in spite of the increased medication, was so intense that he was rarely up from his bed for more than forty-five minutes at a time. He now used his left hand for eating; one evening as we were eating dinner I noticed that his right hand was resting in his serving of cottage cheese—and he was totally unaware of it! There seemed to be no sensation left on that side of his body. He was unable to sleep for more than two or three hours at a time through the night. His system was so filled with chemicals that at least once during the course of each day his body would reject the medications and he would vomit. Food not only did not interest him—it almost nauseated him.

Surprisingly, as this extremely rapid physical decline set in, his spirits seemed to rally. Although for months we had spent endless hours conversing, now as he spent most of his days and evenings lying on his bed, I sat with him in his room and he still found much to talk about.

One afternoon as I was sitting there, looking very sad I suppose, he said, "Hey Mash, you know, you're a very lucky mother."

I said, "Oh, how do you figure that Josh?"

"Well, let's just size up the situation. Here you've had me home for a whole year, all the time, day after day. I don't know how many hours we've spent talking together, but anyway you look at it, if I had not been sick, in a whole lifetime you wouldn't have seen that much of me. After all, young men are off to college, or go away to work, then get married and have their own lives. Yes, any way you look at it Mash, you're a very lucky mother."

The whole week has become a blur of Josh's pain. On Friday, Josh spoke to me for three or four hours, just about his brother. Finally he had me distill all that he had said into a few paragraphs that he wanted Simon to have. I wrote it out and then read it back to him. In essence, he said that Simon was to have everything of his—clothes, the movie camera, any of his other possessions.

Then he gave me a lecture: "Stop pampering Simon. Make him face the responsibility for his behavior, because he's a great kid and he just has to get himself on the right path and he'll be just fine. Don't support him—not if you love him. He's gotta stand on his own two feet—and those size fourteens are solid enough!"

Saturday morning Josh was barely able to rise from his bed to go to the bathroom. His right side was almost totally useless. The pain in his head had now become so excruciating that it actually pushed the back pain from his consciousness. He was writhing in agony. I called Dr. Goldman and finally reached him through his service. All he could offer was more Demarol. It hadn't worked before, and certainly could not work now, but I gave some to Josh. We tried reaching Dr. Stark at UCLA and there was no answer. It had never occurred to us before, but we were so desperate now to respond to Josh's agony that we looked Dr. Stark up in the phone book and, astonishingly, found his home number. He lived not far from us in Santa Monica. I called and a sweet-voiced woman answered, undoubtedly Mrs. Stark. I said, "I'm sorry to intrude but I must speak to the doctor. This is Mrs. Friedman."

She said, "Oh, Josh's mother, just wait a moment please."

Again, one of those flashes of absolute knowledge came to my mind, just as when the secretary had responded with "Oh, poor Josh." I knew that Dr. Stark must have told his wife about the imminence of Josh's death, because she knew immediately who I was although I'd never called before.

I told Dr. Stark that Josh had reached the point where we felt something drastic had to be done. Dr. Stark said, "Don't make a hasty decision. Call me back in a couple of hours."

Just at this time, Ben-Ami arrived unexpectedly. He had heard through the family, during the past few weeks, that Josh's condition was worsening and he decided to fly out for a visit. He and Leib spoke in the living room while I went in to Josh. I brought him more Demarol, four or five of the codeine pills and huge quantities of aspirin. He was taking pills by the handful. It really didn't matter anymore —anything to get some relief.

Josh knew that I had called Dr. Stark and asked me what the doctor had said. I told him and he said, "Mom, please don't do this. Call him back, I have really had it. I cannot explain to you how awful this is and I am so tired. This is all I want. Please do this."

Then he said, "Leave me alone for a little while, please. Let the pills work, let me feel a little better."


*February 24, 1973*

*The hours may be different, but the discussions continue . . . continue. Especially the last two weeks, things are going worse and worse and worse. Man, I am really ruined. I mean every day the last couple of weeks have just been going worse and worse. We just talked to Dr. Stark . . .*

you know, you, me, Mom—I get 'em mixed up. Anyway, we went to the doctor at UCLA and things are worse and worse and worse, now it's the worst. We're so unhappy; it's so true, all the crap that happens. Anyway, I've been so bad, feeling so bad. Things are out of hand. My right hand, it varies, all the way from my foot, from the toe, all the way up to the head. It comes and goes. I'm losing control. Sometimes just no feeling. I wash my hands and everything on the right is just not there. My talking has been going bad . . . bad, too. I'm just not feeling good. Smart fellow, you bet. I started to talk — I have a back . . . My talking— I have a bad lisp sometimes. Now, you see I'm so-so, but with this thing I'm losing control. I talk poorly. 'Cause one side of me I have no sound, no pain but no control. Like I told you, this is like the worst ever. Things have been going so out of hand.

Two or three days ago, the pain—it's bad. This is out of hand. These pains, I don't know why I take it. I could just say, "Come on, just get rid of me somewhere," cause that's how bad it is. It's unbelievable. I just talk — talk so you'll know what it was all about. I'm not pissed at anybody, except myself perhaps. I should do it myself. But now I'm so sick, I can't do it. The last two days, I'm so sick, so painful, you wouldn't believe this. I say, "Oh! help, help." But I can't do it. They'll have to take me over to UCLA or a room and just give me morphine—just finish it off . . . You know I haven't had it yet, don't worry, this is realistic time, I'm not playing. I mean I — We haven't done it yet—but, oh my, it's really ruined my nervousness — I know what I'm trying to say, but your hands are nervous—you feel your hands just brrrrrrrrr . . . I told you that, I told you this. Unbelievable! Plus the headache. I've taken as many Bayer's aspirins—they don't do one bit good at all. I don't know what Mom gave me; in one hour seven of those and they just don't do anything.

The last couple of days, it's so bad, just about the time

262

when let's say, "That's enough, that's enough!" I've had this hell—oh, this pain is unbelievable — I don't think I want to live anymore — I've hit the point, I've hit the point. This pain—ohhh. My hands are so nervous, and my system is just so ruined. I just hope — I have no strength — I just hope . . . I don't know what. Maybe you'll see it and maybe you'll read it and listen to it— Man, I'm in . . . and says she doesn't have any pain. I'm losing my noggins.

It's four-thirty in the afternoon, Saturday. All the stuff in my stomach just keeps on coming up. Now, I'm at the point — I'm saying, "Come on just let me—" This is too much . . . I'm losing everything — maybe it'll come back. Maybe things will be perfect. The words are coming perfect—my explanation is perfect. Everything is perfect. It's there, the pain, but you can fake it. Who knows? I think Mom wants it, I mean, she doesn't even— I mean, I'm getting a little annoyed 'cause that time, when the pains come, I haven't done anything to help. They shouldn't be sorry. They know what's fair is fair.

In addition to the things that I mentioned, sometimes I feel things — sometimes there is no coordination, and I can't feel one side of me. And my head—extremely bad headache — extremely bad headaches . . . Sometimes when I talk, it's hard to explain, but I can't say things, like . . . I kind of talk with a lisp, with a lisp. One side is OK but the other side, no. The eyes—something is wrong with my eyes. They're obviously not right. I don't know—they're certainly not a hundred per cent. If your eyes are normal, you've got a hundred per cent. I don't know, they're obviously less than a . . . ah . . . you know eighty. I don't know exactly what, but they go anywhere from eighty per cent down to like forty per cent. You know, I'm just losing my eyesight. Pressure has something to do with it. Anyway, you know, they were once normal, just normal eyes. Now, they're both losing everything . . . Bad episode.

I saw Sime Thursday. Apparently Saturday there was a

*couple of calls . . . Certainly I've not been feeling good.*
*I guess I'm— Guess my heart, guess my heart goes . . .*
*That's something. I don't know what to talk about.*
*I think I'm here . . . out of hand . . . oh — What's the*
*next? Saw Leib. It is Saturday and he's doing nothing, he's*
*concerned with what's going on with me. I don't know . . .*
*hard to tell . . . recognize. This is, as they say, a fiasco. Boy,*
*one of the fun things that we did, Dad and me, when we*
*were in England, we could . . . like some pretty stupid*
*things. That's a hundred per cent the truth. And that's the*
*truth!* [Here, Josh imitates Lily Tomlin making a "rasp-
berry sound" on *Laugh-In.*] *I'm Laugh-In today. Oh, man!*
*I guess I'll say hello, or good-bye, at the moment. I need*
*something. Some of these drugs you've been giving me,*
*I'll miss. To say the least, they don't solve the answer. And*
*Joshie knows the best. Everything's groovy. I'm losing my*
*mind. I think I really will cut it short now. Good-bye,*
*everybody. See you later!*

I told Leib what Josh had said and a short while later he
called Dr. Stark again. The doctor said, "Bring him to the
hospital this afternoon. I'll arrange for a room."

In the meantime, Ben-Ami stepped in to see Josh for
just a moment or two, but Josh couldn't talk with him. The
pain was too much. Later, I went back into Josh's room.
It was close to four o'clock and the extraordinary number
of pills I had been giving him finally had some effect. The
extreme intensity of his pain was somewhat dulled. Josh
said, "Did you speak to the doctor?"

I told him, "Yes, Dad did. He told Dad that if the pain
is unbearable, if it's all unbearable now, Josh, we can go
to the hospital."

Josh looked at me with absolute trust in his eyes and
asked, "And it will be just three or four days and I'll have
no pain?"

264

"Yes, Josh, that's what the doctor told us."

"Fine, that's just what I want. I've waited too long as it is. Please, I want that now."

I helped him out of bed and he said he wanted to dress to go to the hospital. I said, "Fine, Dad'll help you."

"No, I can manage."

"Well, Dad wants to come in anyway."

Leib went in and he started crying. Josh put his arm around his shoulder and said, "Dad, don't cry, please don't cry. This is the very best thing and I want this. Don't cry, Dad." When Leib came out of the room I went back in and Josh said, "You know, I'm not unhappy, and I don't want you to be unhappy. I want you to be pleased for me because now I won't have to suffer anymore."

"Fine, Josh, fine. I am pleased for you. That's the truth. I don't want you to suffer anymore.

"Remember, Mom, all the times I've talked about this? I'm dying—but you and Dad and Simon are going to live. And you're going to have great times—everything is going to be fine."

I smiled at him and said, "Josh, you're right. We are going to be fine—not to worry."

"Who's worrying, Dim?" Josh responded. "I just want to know what kind of a crazy sports car you're going to get when the bucks start rolling in?" It was an old dream Josh and I shared.

"A Morgan plus two—with belts on the bonnet and wire wheels."

He was laughing now. "And in the garage every other day for tune-ups!"

"Who cares? We'll be rich!" I said.

"And fifty is nifty but eighty is greaty! Just like we always planned, huh Mom?"

"And Joshie, you're gonna be on that seat beside me— all the way, laughing in the wind."

"Old lady, you can count on that" he said, laughing.

We came laughing from his room. Leib was waiting for us in the living room. Josh tried to stoop to pet the cats but couldn't bend. He looked around him and softly said, "Good-bye apartment. So long Tony, fat-cat. 'Bye Coco." Then carrying himself rigidly erect, he walked out of the apartment. His vision was so distorted now that on leaving the apartment, he bumped into the wall of the corridor. He turned to me and smiling ruefully said, "Well, I hope I make it to the hospital without hurting myself."

We went down to the car and drove slowly to the hospital. He would not let me take him upstairs in one of the wheelchairs but insisted on walking like a man to his own death. We went upstairs to the same area where so much of his recent past had been spent. Many of the people there recognized him. Several of the nurses came over to greet him, and one of the male nurses Josh liked helped him undress and get into a hospital gown. This time when we came to the hospital, we hadn't brought pajamas or his medicines—they were no longer necessary.

It was now five-thirty. All the medication I had given Josh at home was starting to wear off, and the pain, in his back and especially in his head, was coming back in waves. As I walked down the corridor to speak with the nurse, I noticed that there was a young Japanese-American doctor sitting in the personnel room having some coffee. I asked a nurse to please get the doctor. Josh had come to the hospital because he needed help for his pain and it was getting worse very rapidly. I asked at five-thirty. We asked again at six and at six-thirty. The pain was mounting.

Finally, at about seven, this same young Japanese-American doctor whom I had seen sitting and drinking coffee came into the room—fully an hour and a half after I had first requested his attention for my son. He was the resident on duty. I told him that Josh was now suffering great pain and we would very much appreciate it if he could arrange to have some morphine brought right away, that we had been waiting now for over an hour. His answer was that they first had to get a medical history. A young intern joined him, and they began a questioning process that lasted almost half an hour.

I was beginning to lose my temper and I said, "Dr. Fukawa, Josh is in great pain. We came to the hospital specifically to get some relief for him from this pain. We did not come in the expectation that you would suddenly develop some miracle cure. This procedure can wait and Josh should be given relief."

He said, "No, I can't prescribe any medicine until the medical examination has been done."

It was close to eight o'clock by now. Josh was writhing on the bed. He said, "Mom, what's going on? I can't stand it . . . you promised no more pain."

I turned to that incredibly insensitive, pompous fool costumed to play the role of healer and insisted that he get some relief to Josh. He told me, "You're just making it worse for him. Until you go out of this room and let me finish my examination there will be no medication." Like puppets being manipulated on strings Leib and I left the room, deserting our son in his agony. There was no excuse for our behavior. I should have been shouting the hospital down while Leib throttled that ego-inflated sadist.

Earlier in the day, before leaving for the hospital, we'd called Simon and explained the situation. A little after eight, Simon came rushing down the hallway. He wanted to know what was happening and we explained.

He looked at us with intense disgust and demanded, "How can you permit them to do this to Josh?"

Simon rushed down the corridor to the telephone and called Dr. Stark. It hadn't even occurred to us. How stupid we were, how mindlessly cruel. Within twenty minutes Dr. Stark came striding down the corridor. We were wait-

267

ing outside of Josh's room. It was close to nine o'clock. We told him that Josh was in terrible pain and they had not yet given him any medication, that we had been there four hours. He went into the room and within moments the intern and the resident issued from the room and slunk down the hall. A few minutes later a nurse came hurrying up with a hypodermic syringe and went into the room.

Dr. Stark came out to speak with us. He was very angry. In a rather loud voice he said, "Josh has been brought to the hospital for treatment. We are not in the business of killing people, we are in the business of saving lives."

I said, "Dr. Stark I know that. All I said to the resident was that we had come here seeking relief from pain."

Dr. Stark said, a bit more quietly, "All right, but it must be understood that if Josh shows improvement, he will be returned to your home."

I know that the purpose of this insane exchange was to establish the fact that he was following procedures—that he could not later be accused of illegal medical activities: Josh's imminent death must be the unfortunate, unanticipated result of "saving" practices. I appreciated his position. I realize that the present legal posture of our hospitals and our medical personnel is such that one cannot openly assist a terminally ill patient to a comfortable and easy death, even when the patient wishes. Therefore, the doctors, the patient, and the family are all forced to play these games. It is a mad and brutal charade, and nobody is really fooled by it. Obviously, if there had been any intention at this point of saving Josh's life, the prime requirement would have been the administering of his regular medications. There was not even a suggestion that these be given to him.

Because these are the archaic rules of the game, although there are innumerable chemicals that could, with one injection, end Josh's suffering and his life, this was not permitted. He, and we, would have to wait until the cumulative effects of the morphine finally impaired his other vital signs, ultimately restricting his breathing and his heart action. But I had not said this out loud because I was aware that it must not be said, nor had Josh said it. Nevertheless, that self-important resident used the authority dangerously misplaced in him to impose the unnecessary cruelty of putting Josh through an agonizingly long medical history and examination. He was playing the game with dirty rules. At any rate, after Dr. Stark established the legality of his position, and I indicated that I completely understood, this was no longer a problem and they could now genuinely address themselves to Josh's needs.

Dr. Stark left. We went into Josh's room. He said he was feeling somewhat better; the nurses had given him an injection of morphine and he was no longer in severe pain. He was just uncomfortable and somewhat apprehensive. "Hey, Mom. What's going to happen—why are they doing this to me?"

I said, "Josh, I'm sorry. There was just a mistake with that doctor, but no more. Dr. Stark was here and they will give you medication when you need it so that you will not have any more pain. We just spoke to him."

He was exhausted from all of the pain, the process of the examination, and the delay in getting the morphine. He said, "All right, I'll rest now."

Feeling confident that Josh would now be free of pain and would be able to sleep, I said, "All right, then we'll go home, Josh. Sleep well, sweetheart. We'll be back in the morning to see you."

It must have been close to ten o'clock when we left the hospital. When we got home, I went in to take a hot bath. At about eleven o'clock, just as I had gotten out of the tub, the telephone rang and I heard Leib answer. It was Josh. He said he was in extreme pain, he had asked the nurse for more medication but she hadn't given him any. It was so bad that he couldn't stand it. He told Leib it was unfair, it was not what had been promised him. Leib, who was still dressed said, "All right, Josh, I'll be right over," and he left immediately for the hospital.

About twelve-thirty Leib returned to the apartment and said that Josh had been very uncomfortable when he got to him. He spoke with the nurse and she checked her chart, or whatever it was that she did, and finally agreed to give Josh another morphine injection. As soon as Josh felt better, Leib left to come home. He hadn't been home long when the phone rang again and I rushed to answer. It was Josh and he said, "It's just awful. My head is killing me and they're not paying attention to me and I can't stand the pain."

Simon couldn't bear this. I had started to dress to go to the hospital and Simon said, "Please Mom, let me go. Let me do this for my brother. There have been so many things I haven't done but this I am going to do. He will not suffer any more tonight." And Simon tore out of the house.

About three o'clock in the morning, Simon was back. He had again done the most logical thing. When he arrived at the hospital close to two o'clock he asked the nurses to give Josh more pain medication and they said no. So he called Dr. Stark. That gracious gentleman responded to this two-o'clock-in-the-morning, semihysterical phone call from Simon with, "Thank you for calling me, Simon. I appreciate you making me aware of this situation and I assure you that it will be immediately attended to." Then Dr. Stark called back the hospital and spoke with the nurses. I do not know what his original orders had been regarding medication, but as of that time, three o'clock in the morning, Josh was to receive morphine injections whenever he felt he needed them. They were to be given on demand. Their frequency was not to be considered. Simon came home feeling that he had rendered a final, crucial service to his brother—and indeed he had.

Early the next morning, we were back at the hospital. Josh had asked us to tell everyone—there were to be no exceptions—that he wanted no one to come to the hospital to see him in his final days. He would permit only Leib, Simon, and me to see him. I could understand his feelings and I felt that they should be honored. We spoke to our relatives and explained the situation to them. We told them that Josh wanted no visitors, that he would prefer that they remember him as he had been at home.

When we arrived at the hospital and got up to Josh's room, he was just being walked back to bed from the bathroom by Ed, one of the male nurses. His vision was almost totally gone. He looked straight at me in the doorway of his room, but I don't think he recognized me until I spoke. The morphine had already been administered in such dosage that his pupils no longer dilated in response to light changes. His eyes were two huge orbs of very pale blue-gray with pinpoint black pupils in the center. Ed got him back into bed and left. I spoke quietly with Josh. Although his eyes could not focus and there was a slight slur in his speech, he was completely conscious and completely cognizant of my being there and of our speaking together. He said he was now getting as much medication as he needed and was only slightly uncomfortable. He had a little headache but otherwise he did not hurt. Shortly thereafter, the same dreadful young resident came into the room, stood beside Josh's bed, took his pulse and blood pressure and then asked Josh, "How are you feeling?"

Josh, unable to focus his eyes and never having known the doctor's name asked, "Are you the Japanese doctor?" It was obviously meant only as a question to determine which doctor was speaking with him. That poor excuse for a doctor, so wrapped up in his own ego, responded to this dying boy with a rather harsh, "I am an American." Moments later, he left the room. Fortunately, we never saw him again. Simon came and saw Josh once again before leaving to return to San Diego. The new semester had just started and he thought he ought to attend classes. There was nothing he could do here, and I agreed that would be best. We were not sure how long this would last. A little later Leib came up; he had brought his mother with him. When Josh was able to perceive that Leib was there with his grandmother, he looked stricken and tried to rise from his bed. I quickly motioned Leib and Adina out of the room, and said, perhaps ungraciously, "Leib, you know what we promised." They realized it had been selfish of her to come despite Josh's express wishes. He still lived— he still had the right to control his life. Leib took her home.

I stayed with Josh until early afternoon when Leib came back. The nurses were now giving Josh medication whenever he requested it. He was still able to press the buzzer attached to his bed to ring for the nurse, but more frequently he would ask me to do it. I tried to feed Josh a bit of the food being served, but he was unable to eat. I held some water for him and he sipped a little. In the afternoon he fell asleep and I told Leib I would go home for a while. I was expecting my parents and I wanted to intercept them at the apartment to stop them from coming to the hospital.

Leib came home late in the afternoon and said that Josh had been dozing on and off since I'd left. He'd had a long talk with the male nurse and had gotten a different insight into this problem of the dying patient. Ed told him that all of the personnel were always aware of the true situation when a patient came into the hospital in this condition. There were strongly divergent opinions among the staff as well as the doctors as to the proper procedure in these cases. Many of the nursing people felt that they could do nothing, they would do nothing, and would consider it not only illegal but immoral to assist in hastening the death of a terminal patient. Others, such as himself, felt that it was not only moral, but almost a requirement of humanity, to do anything in their power to hasten the final agony, to end the suffering. He said we were very fortunate that Josh's doctor was humane, that there were other doctors on the staff who would not grant even this long, drawn-out procedure for easing a person's death, that there were some who would not permit the morphine to exceed absolutely safe levels. The result was a patient in constant agony, never receiving medication in sufficient amounts to counteract the pain; their terminal illnesses even in the most agonizing final stages would be permitted to drag on for weeks. He said that from his previous experience he believed Josh had now suffered his last conscious pain. They had by this time—twenty-four hours after Josh's entry into the hospital—introduced an adequate level of morphine into his system, so that although he might appear slightly fretful, he was no longer experiencing genuine pain. Even the small amount of discomfort he might still be aware of would soon be over.

We went back to the hospital and spoke with Josh. He was, contrary to what the nurse believed, perfectly conscious. He was not in pain when we arrived, but shortly thereafter he said he felt his headache returning. I rang for the nurse and within a moment she was there with another injection. As he could not eat, they had now hung beside his bed, feeding into his arm, the usual intravenous liquid and food supplement. We stayed for an hour or two, until Josh dozed off, and then went home.

At about ten o'clock, I told Leib that I was going back to the hospital. Josh was far from unconscious and I simply could not stand the possibility he might suffer through another night such as the last. That night I spent with Josh, sitting in the chair beside his bed. He dozed only fitfully throughout the night. Whenever he woke, perhaps every thirty minutes, he was lucid. Although he was no longer able to carry on any conversation, each time he would float into wakefulness, he would ask if I was there and clutch my hand. Several times during the night he told me he was uncomfortable. I rang for the nurses and they came quickly with more morphine. Several times during the night I held some water to his lips and he sipped. As the night progressed, he became less wakeful. I am certain, however, that he was fully cognizant all through that endless night that I was there. Every time he woke he would say, "Mom, Mom." I would answer him and he'd slip back into semi-consciousness or sleep, I don't quite know which.

When Leib arrived the next morning at about nine-thirty, I went home and fell asleep. At about two-thirty or three I awoke. Leib had just come back from the hospital. He told me that Josh had had only a few hours of consciousness since morning. He said only one thing to Leib. He tried to indicate to Leib that he was thirsty but Leib didn't understand him. He smiled a little and he said, "Dad, you know your gears and mine never meshed." Then he fell asleep. It was the last thing he ever said.

As the next couple of hours passed Leib realized that Josh was not asleep but was now comatose. Every hour and a half or two, the nurses came and administered more morphine. Josh was almost motionless and seemingly unaware of anything around him.

We went back to the hospital late that afternoon. Josh was indeed comatose. He was perfectly still, completely unresponsive to our presence, totally unaware of the injections he was receiving. That night when we went home I told Leib, "I hope Josh isn't still alive in the morning. It's so pitiful seeing him there so helpless, dying." Leib agreed.

But the next day when we arrived at the hospital Josh was still alive, still comatose. They had moved him to a private room. Throughout this whole, awful period of his final hospitalization, he was perfectly cared for—always fresh linens, clean and pure-looking. In addition to the bottle that was feeding into the veins of his arm, there was a catheter leading from under his bedsheet to a waste collection bottle and I noticed that there was some blood in the urine. His system was starting to break down. We saw Dr. Stark that day. He gave me a gentle lecture on not staying there day and night. I told him, "No, no, I just stayed that one night because Josh was still conscious and there was value in doing it. On the contrary, we are very calm now, and very accepting. We only wish that Josh won't have much longer to go through this."

Dr. Stark said, "Yes, I know how you feel but he is in no pain. He feels nothing, he knows nothing, it will not be long."

Wednesday back at the hospital there seemed to be no change. His pulse was still strong and his breathing regular. The only difference was that there was a phlegmy sound to his breathing. I asked the nurse about it and she said they periodically cleared the mucus by suction. I suppose in response to my question, she proceeded to force a rubber tube down his throat to remove the fluid collections. Josh made almost no response to this awful treatment. He was no longer sentient.

When we returned home Wednesday evening I felt that there would still be a long, awful wait. Josh seemed so strong. As usual, I couldn't fall asleep. At about three in the morning, for the first time during all the months of Josh's illness, I decided to take some sleeping pills to get some respite from this agonizing process of thinking, waiting, and watching for his death. At five-thirty Leib was shaking me awake. As a result of the sleeping pills I had not even heard the telephone ring. I was very foggy from the pills. Leib was shaking me by the shoulders, shaking me. Then, swimming into awareness, I heard him say, "Mash, our son is dead!"

We got dressed immediately. I tried to clear my head. I was totally awake but I felt waves of nausea from the barbiturates. It was Thursday morning, March 1, 1973. We reached the hospital about an hour after Josh's death. He was lying in that private, quiet, dim room where we had seen him the day before. They had changed his hospital gown and had put fresh linens on the bed. He was beautifully clean and calm and peaceful. A nurse was sitting beside his bed. When we came in, she stepped out of the room to leave us alone with the body of our son.

A miracle had occurred. I suppose as a result of the cessation of the cortisone he had been taking, all the puffiness that he had in his face for all those months was gone. Because he was so thin, he looked beautifully ascetic. Since the blood had stopped pounding through his body, the acne discolorations that had looked so grotesque on his face were gone; his skin was perfect, as it had been for all of his life before his illness. I don't know what happened so soon after his death. I don't know if fluid had discharged from all the cells in his body, but by some incredible physiological process, that obscene protrusion on the side of his head had subsided and the flap had settled itself into a normal position. Josh, lying there peacefully, was again the handsome youth he had been before the entire horror started. Only the ivory color of his skin suggested death rather than sleep.

I bent over and kissed his cheek. He was cold. He was dead.

# Epilogue

Fear not death; we are destined to die. We
share it with all who ever lived, with all
who ever will be. Bewail the dead,
hide not your grief, do not restrain your
mourning. But remember that continuing
sorrow is worse than death. When the
dead are at rest, let their memory rest,
and be consoled when the soul departs.

Apocrypha, Ben Sira 41:13, 38:17–23

After the memorial service for Josh, people said how brave, how stoical we were. There was no other behavior possible; anything else would have dishonored his memory. But the brave face of daylight dissolves in the black hours of night and there is a shouting in the heart for answers that don't come.

Did we do the right things? Were our decisions the correct ones? We trusted the doctors. I must believe that when they decided to operate they really thought Josh could be cured, that his tumor was not malignant. Any other thought would lead to madness. How many times Josh said he would so happily have taken the few months they said he had and be spared the disfigurement and incapacity of the surgery and what followed. A few months as a whole Josh. And perhaps then the treatment in Japan —and life. And why is that treatment unavailable here? And what of the diagnostic techniques? Why are they so unreliable? Why are we led to believe they are accurate and precise? And what causes these tumors? And why him? *Why?*

Josh is dead; the ashes of his body are scattered at sea. This I know. But I cannot believe it. Can it be possible that Josh will never finish his life, the life just barely started? Never do a man's work, never marry, never be a father, never grow old?

A sea of depression and black despair. Nothing is real except his nonexistence. Do I weep for his death? No, that is too cruel. I must rejoice for him that his pain is ended. Do I weep for myself? How unfair to the memory of his courage. People try to help. Expressions of sympathy— "Time cures all," "You must go on for Simon," endless well-intentioned bromides. Finally, a glimmer of light. A friend, herself childless, reminds me of what I have forgotten. "You dwell on the years you'll be without him. Why don't you remember that you were privileged to enjoy him for twenty-one years?" Of course.

For ninety-five per cent of his life Josh was a wonderful boy—bright, beautiful, loving and loved. For five per cent of his life Josh was a magnificent man. I was indeed privileged to be his mother. The real loss would be not to have had him at all.

Unbidden, like flashbacks in movies, I see in my mind pictures of Josh. They come with great frequency. Visions of Josh dead, riding his bike, playing tennis, lying in bed to ease his pain, laughing, coming from school, playing Scrabble, dead. It is not sad, because only thus can I ever again see him. I would exchange the balance of my years to touch him again—impossible wish. Death is irreversible and only his absence is tangible.

There is something fundamentally improper and at variance with nature for parents to outlive their grown children.

Death is the one certainty we are all guaranteed at birth. But there are rules even for death—and their abrogation is what creates tragedy.

Man knows, with atavistic certitude, that babies in their frailty and purity and susceptibility may sicken and die. Young men, in their lusty vitality and aggressive strength, test fate and sometimes lose. They die violently, in accident and in war, shaking their fists in the face of danger and challenging circumstance to break their pulsating power in one great explosion of energy. The natural rules do not provide for a young man to suffer a slow, debilitating, agonizing, irreversible illness and death. That is an old man's way to die. Old bodies wear out and deteriorate, but in the intervening years, before that happens, one has time to learn patience and acceptance, time to define one's relationship to infinity.

Courage, like love and dignity, has never been adequately defined. Perhaps the only definition of these concepts lies in example and, although we cannot say what they are, we recognize them when they are manifest. My son was courage, love and dignity. I do not know what mysterious, hidden inner source he tapped for that endless year, but the wellspring never ran dry. He taught those of us willing to learn how to die. We must teach ourselves to live with this unbearable loss.

# Postscript

In June, 1974, we were officially notified that the UCLA Medical Center, in conjunction with the surgeon, had re-evaluated our financial situation. Taking into account the enormous debts we had incurred during Josh's illness, they decided on their own initiative to reduce substantially the balance of the medical bill still outstanding. We are indeed grateful to them.